THE HEALTH CARE MESS

Julius B. Richmond, M.D.

Rashi Fein, Ph.D.

THE HEALTH CARE MESS

HOW WE GOT INTO IT

AND

WHAT IT WILL TAKE

TO GET OUT

HARVARD UNIVERSITY PRESS

Cambridge, Massachusetts, and London, England · 2005

Library of Congress Cataloging-in-Publication Data

Richmond, Julius B. (Julius Benjamin), 1916–
    The health care mess : how we got into it and what it will
    take to get out / Julius B. Richmond and Rashi Fein ;
    foreword by Jimmy Carter.
        p. cm.
    Includes bibliographical references and index.
    ISBN 0-674-01924-5 (alk. paper)
    1. Medical care—United States.   2. Medical policy—
United States.   3. Health planning—United States.
I. Fein, Rashi.   II. Title.

RA395.A3R53 2005
362.1'0973—dc22   2005040396

To Jean and Ruth

Acknowledgments

It is impossible to list all of the people to whom we are indebted for help on this book. They certainly include members of our families who, among other things, adjusted their and our schedules so that we could give priority to this effort. They also include those with whom, over the years, we have discussed the issues raised in these pages and those whose articles and books have helped stimulate our thinking. We also thank our colleagues in the Department of Social Medicine at Harvard Medical School who followed the development of this book with interest, and especially Leon Eisenberg, with whom we have participated in numerous stimulating conversations over the years.

Nevertheless, we can single out a number of those who helped bring this book to completion. The Robert Wood Johnson Foundation provided financial support. Becca Hubble was an invaluable research assistant; this book would not exist without her contribution. Marcia Feldman typed many of the drafts, and Sue Thompson provided important assistance.

A number of our colleagues read drafts of the manuscript. We especially want to thank Allan Brandt, who found the time amid his many responsibilities to make numerous comments and force us to sharpen our discussion and justify our approach and analyses. Steve Berger, Gordon Harper, Michael Heisler, George Lamb, George Lundberg, and David Mechanic also commented and encouraged us to consider additional subjects. Naturally, we alone are responsible for remaining errors of commission and omission.

We wish to thank Harvard University Press and its talented staff members. What began as a somewhat casual conversation with Michael Aronson led to an enjoyable further involvement with Ann

Downer-Hazell who, among her many talents, had the ability to look beyond the raw product we handed her and imagine the finished manuscript. Her colleague Sara Davis was quick to respond to our inquiries and was of great assistance. We are also indebted to Mary Ellen Geer, who saw the manuscript through the various stages that transformed it into a book and did so most effectively. Richard Audet edited the manuscript with great skill. We (and the readers) owe him our thanks.

Contents

Foreword

JIMMY CARTER

When I was President, I wrestled with the twin problems of rapidly rising health care expenditures and the millions of uninsured and underinsured Americans. Over the years since I left office, these problems have gotten worse. Our nation seems even further away from dealing with these threats to the physical, mental, and financial health of all Americans.

I am pleased, therefore, to see this book by two distinguished students of American health care. One of them, Julius Richmond, served ably in my administration as Surgeon-General and Assistant Secretary for Health, and has continued to be my esteemed adviser. Doctors Richmond and Fein have written a book for all of us who have been striving to bring care within the reach and means of all our people. It is rich in historical perspective on why the United States has greatly advanced medical science, but has yet to achieve what all other developed nations have attained: comprehensive health services for all citizens.

At times, the story told in this book reawakens deeply frustrating memories for me. I campaigned for office believing that the health care system needed drastic reorganization. I wanted to lower expenditures by placing a greater emphasis on preventive medicine, outpatient care, priority attention to infants and young children, and cost containment. I also committed myself to creating a national health insurance program and seeing that services were available for people in remote and disadvantaged areas of our country. My proposal would have provided "catastrophic" coverage for all citizens and comprehensive coverage for children up to five years of age, with future expansion. Some congressional and labor leaders considered this inadequate, so no proposal was adopted. Perhaps we have reached the point where a new coalition for reform can be achieved. We have a health system that is deeply frustrating to patients, physicians, and other health professionals, as well as to all those in the private and public sectors who pay higher and higher premiums and allocate larger and larger budgets for ever more restricted coverage. This book helps us understand the strengths of our system as well as what is wrong with it. Most important, it offers a design for a realistic program that would move us forward.

Introduction

There is a disconcertingly large gap, more correctly a chasm, between the scientific glories of American medicine and the delivery failures of the American health care system. The same newspapers that report the latest laboratory and clinical findings and hold out hope for new and more effective therapies also tell us about a dysfunctional insurance system, about the 45 million Americans who, without health insurance, receive less health care and have no protection against the financial impact of illness, and about the anger and irritation of patients, physicians, legislators, and others who encounter or fund American medicine.

We do not believe that the "mess" we are in is preordained. Neither do we believe that it is self-correcting. The American health care system, the way our nation pays for care and organizes it, can be changed in fundamental ways, but only if we choose to do so. Purposeful intervention to increase the effectiveness of our delivery system and to make it more equitable requires the application of enlightened public and private policy. In turn, the policies we select require that we understand how we got here. We need a richer knowledge base. We also need the political will to apply that knowledge and adopt appropriate social strategies for changing our health care system.

We, the co-authors of this book, are optimistic. Part, though by no means all, of that optimism is generated by the vigor and resilience of our health care institutions. Part is generated by the strength of our science and technology base and the opportunities it presents for future progress. Ultimately, however, our optimism derives from our knowledge of the qualities and commitments of the thousands of students who, imbued with idealism and the desire to help others, are studying to become health professionals, the millions of people who work within the health sector, and the tens of millions of Americans who deserve and want a better system. We hope that this book will provide them all with a better understanding of "how we got here," the possibilities and policy options that lie before us, the formidable obstacles we will encounter, and what we must do to avoid further deterioration in the distribution of health care and to enable us to attain an equitable distribution of that care while continuing our scientific advances and making them more accessible.

We believe that those options cannot be fully understood without reference to the past. Where we are at present is influenced by conscious and deliberate choices made in earlier years and, moreover, by choices made without full awareness of their significance, implications, and potential unintended consequences. Nevertheless, our future will not unfold in some deterministic manner in which we are simply bystanders, governed entirely by earlier events and persons whose names, once legend, are today hardly known. We can choose. Our choices, however, are constricted; we cannot ignore our medical, social, and political history and imagine that we are beginning with a *tabula rasa*. History is relevant.

This book, therefore, traces developments in education for medicine and public health and in health care financing and organization over the last century. We pay special attention to the last third of the century, the years following the enactment of Medicare and Medicaid. That emphasis derives from the fact that that period witnessed the century's most "revolutionary" changes in the organization and financing of the delivery of health care. These changes have altered the environment in which health professionals are educated and medicine is practiced. In earlier periods when medicine was expanding its ability to help individuals in distress, we could assume that a growing economy and strong social fabric would enable more and more Americans to benefit from medicine's advances. We can no longer make that assumption. The number of Americans without insurance is growing, not declining. The distribution of income is becoming less equal. The social fabric, the sense of community, appears weaker. These trends and the actions we can take to alter the direction of our health care system are the focus of our inquiry. In writing about American medicine the word "American" is crucially important. We can learn from other countries that have achieved universal coverage, but our delivery and financing systems are "our" systems; American institutions of medical education are "our" institutions. Medicine is not an abstraction; it is rooted in time and place. Our medical schools reflect our higher education structures and their values; our research establishment has been molded by the interplay between the priorities of the National Institutes of Health (and its support for basic science) and the priorities of the private sector (and its emphasis on bringing products to market). Our health care delivery institutions have been influenced by an American ambivalence about the proper roles for government and the market. We have responded to the continuing increase in national health expenditures with conflicting efforts to regulate and to foster free-market competition. Our reliance on the latter makes us unique among industrial countries. All these characteristics, and more, require that we tell an American story that makes reference to political structures and competing values and to views about individual and collective responsibility. Put simply, the study of medicine requires the study of the world exogenous to medicine.

This book is the product of a joint effort. Our long history of collaboration has had an important impact on the perspective of this volume. We both came to Washington, where we first met, in the early 1960s to assume very different responsibilities. Julius Richmond, educated as a physician, developed and was the first head of Head Start, which benefited 23 million children over the next forty years, and Neighborhood Health Centers, both vital programs in the War on Poverty. Rashi Fein, educated as an economist, served on the staff of President Kennedy's Council of Economic Advisers with responsibilities for the analysis of programs and for legislative initiatives in various social and economic areas, importantly including health. After our years in Washington we both returned to academia and some time later crossed paths once again at Harvard Medical School. During the 1970s

Dr. Fein began a long association with Senator Edward Kennedy and the Committee for National Health Insurance, thereby furthering his involvement with the legislative branch of government. In the mid-1970s Dr. Richmond returned to Washington to serve in President Carter's administration as Assistant Secretary for Health in the Department of Health, Education, and Welfare and as Surgeon-General in the United States Public Health Service.[1] Subsequently, we resumed our association at Harvard while maintaining our connections to government and private sector policy formulation. That made possible countless hours of conversation about health policy and the directions that the nation's health care system was taking. Though we came with different backgrounds and out of different fields, both of us brought the outlook of the academic and the policy maker and adviser. We have lived in both arenas, and our attitudes and the framework and insights of this book are informed by our multiple roles and experiences.

Both of us share a view about our country. We deplore the wide disparities not only in health care but in income, education, housing, and other important factors that affect well-being and opportunity. We especially believe in the importance of enhancing the development of young children. We are confident that through effective public policy we can build a more equitable community in which many more of our neighbors would be able, not only to dream the American dream, but to fulfill it. We have both been involved in efforts to bring more equity to health care delivery because of our conviction that health and health care are vitally important in influencing life's chances and that one's income and wealth should not determine the amount and quality of care one receives. We seek a system in which the financing and distribution of health services reflect our image of a just society, a society in which economic arrangements reflect a moral dimension. We hope that our book will help revive the debate about how to proceed toward the goal of equitable health care.

We have used the term "revolution" in describing various periods and developments in medical education and medical care. We should be clear: what we call revolutions do not begin on a given date and end later at some fixed time. Rather, they involve the gradual emergence of new patterns of thought and action. Thus each revolution blends with the past and, in turn, continues to influence subsequent periods. Gradually the newer issues and attitudes take over and come to dominate, having absorbed the legacy of the revolution that came before. Although the revolutions we write about involve large changes, they appear as revolutions only in retrospect.

The first two chapters of our volume discuss what may be termed "the coming of age of American medicine." These set the scene for the drama that emerges in the last third of the century. The first chapter discusses the changes that took place in education and in science beginning in the early decades of the century, changes that enabled medicine to do more in a more effective manner for more people. As a consequence of medicine's growing abilities and successes, access to and the availability of medical care assumed increasing importance. This topic is explored in the second chapter, in which we discuss the development and expansion of health insurance in the United States and the enactment of Medicare and Medicaid in 1965. In Chapters 3 and 4 we examine the reactions to the implementation of Medicare, the federal social insurance program that provides health insurance to those age sixty-five and over and (since 1973) the disabled, as well as Medicaid, the state and federal program that pays for health care for many (but not all) of the poor. We look at the impact of the burgeoning health sector on expenditures, on the regulatory attempts to control their growth, and on education for the health professions.

As a consequence of the failure of regulatory efforts to control expenditures, the body politic turned to the free market in the hope that competitive forces would rein in the growth of the health sector as a share of all economic activity. Chapters 5 and 6 examine the impact of this development with special attention to the implications of the expansion of for-profit institutions and their role in the delivery of medical care services, the increasing intrusion of for-profit investment criteria into medical care decisions, and the new entrepreneurial ethos with which the organized health professions could not cope. Throughout the various chapters we pay special attention to the efforts to enact legislation that would provide health insurance to all Americans and to enhance the equitable distribution of health care.

In Chapters 7 and 8 we discuss the challenges and opportunities the nation faces at the present time. Chapter 7 focuses on medicine and medical education. The probability of important advances is great, and the public can look forward to new therapies and more effective care. Chapter 8 turns to the question whether these substantial advances will be available to a public among whom the number of uninsured individuals is increasing year by year and for whom we have not yet erected a substitute for our employment-linked health insurance system that is weakening and at risk. The chapter focuses on equity and universal health insurance. We are convinced that our delivery system is in crisis, and without some intervention, private sector insurance will continue to leave an increasing number of our fellow citizens without insurance and without appropriate care. We examine the criteria that should guide efforts to develop a universal health program and offer our own proposal to accomplish that goal.

Part I

THE EARLY YEARS
(1900–1965)

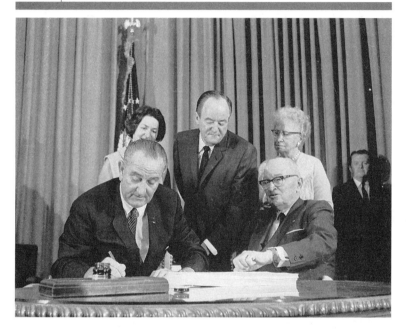

Former President Harry S Truman checks the exact time as President Lyndon Baines Johnson signs Medicare, the last major legislation enacted in health care, on July 30, 1965, with their two wives and Vice President Hubert H. Humphrey looking on. Photograph © Bettmann/CORBIS.

1 The Educational and Scientific Revolution: Higher Standards and Changing Priorities

Scientific advances taking place in the early twentieth century were destined to have a significant impact on diagnostic and therapeutic interventions available to physicians, the understanding of disease patterns, and the nature of medical education and physician preparation for the emerging modes of practice. Discoveries in the natural sciences and the increasing availability and applications of the compound microscope fostered the development of pathology, bacteriology, physiology, pharmacology, and biochemistry as sciences basic to the study of medicine. The development of x-ray examinations, electrocardiography, and laboratory examinations of body fluids, based on new knowledge in physics and chemistry, were beginning to change the nature of medical practice.

It has been said that, at the turn of the last century, if a randomly selected patient with a random illness met a randomly selected physician, the patient had only a fifty-fifty chance of benefiting from the encounter. Those odds increased remarkably over the century, and that increase began in the early decades.

The Educational Revolution and the Rise of the Guild Establishment

One hundred years ago medical education took place in a large number of schools, many of which were privately owned and few of which were associated with institutions of higher education. These schools produced a great many physicians who met the then-prevailing standards. As a consequence America had a favorable physician-population ratio and a reasonable urban-rural physician distribution. Had there not been a shift in medicine's science base, existing schools and American medical education would have felt little pressure to change. But science was advancing and change was in the air.[1] Few of the existing proprietary schools had or could obtain the resources to upgrade and expand their faculty and facilities (especially their laboratories), or develop relationships to teaching hospitals and provide richer clinical and laboratory instruction, thereby encompassing the developments in science. It seemed impossible and much too costly to improve all existing schools (even presuming that there had been a sufficient number of qualified faculty and students to do so). Nor did it seem desirable to maintain existing educational patterns while gradually developing new curricula and raising standards of education and performance a few schools at a time and over a lengthy period. The question, therefore, was how to proceed, and the answer was not at all obvious.

As a consequence of its interest in professional education in general and with the cooperation of the Council on Medical Education of the American Medical Association (AMA) assured, the Carnegie Foundation for the Advancement of Teaching prevailed upon Abraham Flexner, a distinguished educator, to survey the state of medical education in the United States and Canada and to make recommendations for its improvement. Issued in 1910, the Flexner Report is recognized as one of the most important developments in American medical education, research, and service.[2] In due course the advances in science most probably would have had their impact on medical education even without a Flexner Report; nevertheless, there is little doubt that the report speeded and provided a template for change. It encouraged the adoption of a four-year medical school curriculum, introduced laboratory teaching exercises, improved the quality of instruction through a full-time faculty, expanded clinical teaching through the introduction of the clinical clerkship, brought medical schools into the framework of the universities, and—rejecting the pattern, common in many countries, of separation of research programs into institutes—incorporated research into medical school teaching programs.

The adoption of the changes that Flexner called for was facilitated by grants from the General Education Board of the Rockefeller Foundation, which from 1910 to 1928 distributed seventy-eight million dollars among the medical schools of twenty-four universities. This rapid response and adoption of the major recommendations offer further evidence that medical education leaders were ready for change and that the Flexner Report provided the catalytic agent. Nevertheless, as so often happens, yesterday's changes become tomorrow's rigidities. It does not detract from the quality of the report to note that this too was the inevitable result of Flexner's recommendations—in part because the proposals could be accomplished only by introducing institutional accreditation criteria and processes and practitioner licensing or certification.

The Association of American Medical Colleges (AAMC), an organization established in 1876 and made up of institutional members of the medical schools, developed a standard curriculum that it incorporated in its by-laws as a requirement for membership. Furthermore, the AMA Council on Medical Education included the curriculum in its statement of essentials of an approved medical school, which in turn served as the basis for accreditation. At the same time the licensing requirements of the various states, expressed through statutes, were patterned on the recommendations of the AAMC and the AMA. Often these described and prescribed the curriculum in considerable detail (even to minimum hours of instruction in individual subjects). Once adopted, these, now institutionalized, standards and requirements could not easily be altered. Inevitably, they led to the demise of many schools.

It should be noted that the AMA Council adopted these quite radical changes even though many of its members had graduated from the very schools that the new accreditation process would eliminate. This behavior may be attributed to "enlightenment" and concern about the quality of education and, therefore, of health care. Conversely, cynics (or are they realists?) might attribute it to early recognition of the economic benefits of guild-like behavior. There is, after all, a long history in which "quality" standards are used to provide a rationale for the restriction of supply.

As a consequence of the institutionalization of Flexner's recommendations, there was a sharp downturn in the number of medical schools and in the number of graduates. In 1906, the peak year, there were 162 schools; by 1910, when the Flexner Report was published, the number had already dropped to 131. In the next twenty years it fell to 76, and some twenty years later still stood at only 79. Similarly, the number of graduates, which peaked at 5,747 in 1904 and which had already declined to 4,440 by 1910, continued its fall and totaled 3,047 in 1920. As late as 1950 it had not yet reached the earlier 1904 figure (though, of course, the 1950 graduate was far better educated than the physician of half a century earlier). The falloff in the number of graduates together with the increase in population resulted in a very substantial decline in the ratio of physicians to population. The 1906 ratio of 158 physicians per 100,000 population fell to 126 in 1931 (a drop of 20 percent) and had hardly risen (to 136) some thirty years later.[3] The unanimous attribution of only good consequences to the Flexner Report, therefore, appears to be somewhat uncritical. It does not ask whether the quality-improvement goals might have been approached by a slower process of attrition that would have had less impact on the availability of care to persons who needed it and who, in subsequent years, had to confront the "doctor shortage."

The AMA and Public Policy

The raising of standards and subsequent decline in the number of M.D. graduates and in the physician-population ratio had an additional important impact. It can be argued that it led the membership of the AMA, increasingly aware of the economic benefits of a tight supply of physicians, to look inward, to adopt guild-like behavior, and increasingly to devote its attention and efforts to what it discerned were the economic interests of its members. During the earliest part of the century and even as late as the second decade, the AMA had allied itself with the American Association for Labor Legislation and others who urged state action to extend health insurance to the population. Thus, for example, a 1917 report of the AMA Committee on Social Insurance recommended that the profession cooperate in efforts to formulate health insurance legislation. That, however, was the last such report. By the mid-1920s, under pressure from state medical societies, the

AMA still spoke of the health of the people, but behaved as if its priority was the health of the profession.[4] Any chance that this change could be reversed disappeared with the trauma of the Great Depression of the 1930s when many physicians were not fully employed, and the profession faced economic problems not dissimilar from those faced by the rest of the population. Furthermore, the depression years were followed by World War II, a period when military service again meant that many physicians had limited incomes. The impact on the medical profession of the period 1930–1945, a full fifteen years of constraints on income, cannot be overestimated. The "protectionist" attitudes formed then came to dominate the patterns of thought of the membership and leadership of organized medicine for many years.

As noted, the forces of conservatism in American organized medicine had already manifested themselves by the 1920s, when America sought "normalcy," and before the trauma of the depression. Since the AMA seemed out of step with those who were concerned about the health needs of the population, eight private foundations turned away from organized medicine and helped establish the Committee on the Costs of Medical Care (CCMC) in 1927. This committee of fifty distinguished individuals was drawn from a broad array of fields: medicine, public health, sociology, economics, and so forth. In the period between 1928 and 1932 the commission and its staff published twenty-eight reports. In October 1932 it adopted its final report, which in many important respects was visionary.[5] Indeed, it was so far ahead of its time that thirty-eight years later, in 1970, the United States Department of Health, Education, and Welfare republished the final report, not as some quaint historical document, but with a preface that stated that the old problems remain and that "now is the time for action!"[6]

The Committee recommended that medical services should be furnished largely by groups of physicians, dentists, nurses, pharmacists, and other associated personnel, preferably organized around a hospital, and that suitable hospitals be developed into comprehensive community medical centers in which the medical professions and the public would participate in the provision of, and the payment for, all health and medical care. The Committee also recommended the provision of requisite funds to enable the extension of all basic public health services—whether provided by governmental or nongovernmental agencies—so that they would be available to the entire population according to its needs. Importantly, while not precluding fee-for-service payment to physicians, it urged that the costs of medical care be placed on a group payment basis, through the use of insurance and/or taxation. It further recommended that the study, evaluation, and coordination of medical service be considered important functions for every state and local community, that agencies be formed to exercise these functions, and that the coordination of rural with urban services receive special attention.

The Committee further recommended that the training of physicians devote larger emphasis to the teaching of health and the prevention of disease, more effective efforts be made to provide trained health officers, the social aspects of medical practice be given greater attention, specialties be restricted to those specially qualified, and postgraduate educational opportunities be increased. There were additional recommendations about professional education in other fields concerned with health care: dentistry, pharmacy, nursing, nursing aides, nurse-midwives, and hospital and clinical administrators.

One wonders what impact the Committee would have had if its report had been issued at a different time, that is, not a short month before the 1932 election when a fearful nation's attention was riveted on economic matters. In 1932 there simply was no venue in which the report could receive the consideration that it was due, no legislative body that, given the crisis the nation faced, had the time to address the CCMC recommendations. Nevertheless, ever-vigilant in guarding against change, the *Journal of the American Medical Association (JAMA)* editorialized that there were two camps: "on the one side [are] the forces representing the great foundations, public health officialdom, social theory—even socialism and communism—inciting to revolution." On the other was a small and lonely band, "the organized medical profession of this country."[7]

The AMA's conservative stance did not change after the depression and the Second World War. The passage of time brought little significant alteration to the political culture of the organization. It is true

that in the 1960s the AMA adopted far less rigid positions on expansion of medical education. Nevertheless, as a consequence of the fragmentation of American medicine and within the AMA, control of the organization remained in the hands of, what can be termed, an "old guard."
This fragmentation and change in priorities stemmed from various factors and took multiple forms. Several influences tended to point the AMA's scientific and professional leadership in a different direction from its practicing physician leadership and its political agenda. For the scientific leadership the professionalization of medical education increasingly received the highest priority. It no longer was acceptable to deliver a series of lectures and thereby discharge one's obligations to students. Laboratory and clinical instruction had to receive more attention and became more and more demanding. A second force for fragmentation stemmed from the theoretical and methodological advances in the sciences that led to a corollary expansion of the research enterprise. As clinical investigation developed more structure and became more complex, a corps of full-time clinical investigators developed. Though they were Doctors of Medicine, they had an allegiance to their scientific disciplines in the university as well as to their clinical disciplines within the medical community.
Concomitant with the growth of scientific knowledge and clinical investigation was the emergence of specialization. Although not averse to dealing with organizational tasks, the scientific leaders in the specialties were not especially active in the AMA. Instead, from the 1920s on, they went about forming their own "academies" and "colleges" and did so with considerable energy and enthusiasm. The various "sections" of the AMA might have served their purpose, but the scientists' political agenda (that called for more resources for research) was far removed from that which drew the attention of practicing physicians and was represented in the councils of the AMA. The new specialty organizations were primarily concerned with the advancement, strengthening, and professionalization of science and education and only secondarily with broad public policy issues, while the AMA was becoming preoccupied with political issues that related to the status, well-being, and interests of practicing physicians.

At the same time medical schools were beginning to manifest their own organizational autonomy. As noted, after the Flexner Report, the Association of American Medical Colleges that had served as little more than a clearing house for information among the medical schools was drawn into the process of accreditation of medical schools in collaboration with the Council on Medical Education of the AMA. Since the AAMC's interest in medical education was quite different from the concerns of the AMA, medical school leaders devoted their energies to the organization that represented their interests and to their own agendas. As a consequence the AMA largely lost the perspectives and contributions that medical educators might have provided.

The large organizational structure of the AMA, although appearing to assure a democratic process, did not provide congenial auspices for the growth of these new or newly active professional organizations. Furthermore, it was clear that the political structure of the AMA made it extraordinarily unlikely that the organization would change. There was only a limited turnover of members of the Board of Trustees in any one year, and the process of election to the Board required the backing of county and state medical societies whose leadership, because of staggered terms of office, also changed only slightly in any single year.

For the individual physician the climb up the organizational ladder in the AMA (from the county through the district and state societies, the House of Delegates, and perhaps finally to the Board of Trustees) was arduous and time-consuming. This sequence resulted in a Board of Trustees whose members generally were over sixty years of age and who had reached their positions because of their conservative views, a situation that contributed to the adoption of policies oriented to the past or to the status quo. As we shall see, over time this had the unfortunate effect of inducing the organization that, at most, spoke for practicing physicians (though it claimed to speak for American medicine) to become a "nay-sayer," an association that was out of step with both Republican and Democratic administrations and legislators who were trying to solve emerging and long-standing problems. In turn, the AMA became marginalized and less relevant to the discussions about appropriate ways to advance the nation's health. America lost the medical community's potential contribution.

During this period in which medical schools were devoting increased attention to the improvement and expansion of their teaching and research facilities and programs they engaged in few innovative or exploratory programs in delivering medical care. Individual faculty members assisted in providing services to low-income people in teaching hospitals and clinics, but the schools did not view the provision of care (or matters concerning its quality) as falling within their responsibility. Similarly, the relatively few schools of public health were oriented toward the teaching of epidemiology and public health administration with relatively little emphasis on medical care financing, organization, or administration. This orientation reflected the general concern of public health officials with the prevailing problems of sanitary engineering and infectious disease control. Regrettably, it left little room for new priorities that would have examined the barriers to the efficient and equitable provision of care.

Nor did public health officials address the topics that the various branches and levels of government were beginning to wrestle with as medical interventions became more effective and questions of availability of, and access to, health care services came to the fore. As a consequence, when medical care legislation was enacted, federally sponsored and funded programs that dealt with the provision and administration of medical services were located in agencies outside the United States Public Health Service (USPHS). For example, the first major medical care programs (enacted as part of the Social Security Act of 1935), authorizing grants to the states for maternal and child health and crippled children's programs, were placed in the United States Children's Bureau. Similarly, in 1950 when the Social Security amendment for vendor (fee-for-service) payments under Public Assistance was enacted, responsibility was not placed in health departments, but in the federal Welfare Administration and state and local welfare offices. Likewise, in 1965, Medicare became part of the Social Security Administration and Medicaid was located in the Welfare Administration. The fact that these health programs were not housed in the USPHS speaks volumes about the limited involvement of the medical community in the broad issues of access to and delivery of care. It speaks volumes as well about the perspective of legislators and federal administrators who (perhaps as a consequence of organized medicine's posture) did not view these programs as health programs but, simply, as cash or in-kind transfer programs.

Nevertheless, it would be a significant error to imply that the medical community had a monolithic view throughout the pre–World War II period (or, for that matter, in the period following the war). Just as with the CCMC, there were important voices that called for a vigorous attack on the nation's health problems. The American Foundation Studies in Government reflected this in a study that collected physicians' opinions.[8] The AMA's lack of interest in and neglect of the report led in 1937 to the organization of a Committee of Physicians, popularly known as the "Committee of 430" because of the number of distinguished physicians who initially sponsored the statement of principles and proposals. The principles of the Committee were stated in forthright fashion: that (1) the health of the people was a direct concern of the government; (2) a national public health policy directed toward all groups within the population should be formulated; (3) the problem of economic need and the problem of providing adequate medical care were not identical and might require different approaches for their solution; and (4) the provision of adequate medical care for the population required the participation of four groups: voluntary agencies, and local, state, and federal government.[9]

An editorial in the *Journal of the American Medical Association* forcefully expressed the AMA's opposition to the opinions of the physicians and to the Committee. The editorial did not simply take issue with the principles that had been enunciated at the formation of the Committee (and with its proposals); it impugned the individuals who supported them:

Obviously some of these men must have signed merely after seeing the names of those who signed previously and because it looked like a "good" list. There appear also the names of some members of the House of Delegates [of the AMA] which voted against some of the very propositions which these members here support. Most conspicuous on the list are the names of those deans and heads of departments in medical schools who may have signed because they saw a possibility of getting government money for clinics and dispensaries.

Such careless participation in propaganda as has here occurred is lamentable, to say the least. Certainly the unthinking endorsers of the American Foundation's principles and proposals owe to the medical profession some prompt disclaimers.[10]

The attack on the Committee and the harassment of individual Committee members reflected increasingly doctrinaire positions that were evolving in the AMA. These attacks, the lack of a staff and organizational base, the informal manner in which the Committee was organized, in addition to a preoccupation with the military mobilization, led to the gradual disappearance of this courageous group. Nevertheless, its members pointed the way toward changes that were to develop following World War II.

Specialization, the Scientific Revolution, and the Rise of the Academic Establishment

Beginning earlier, but especially during the 1930s when nineteen boards in the medical specialties were established, it became increasingly apparent that advances in the medical sciences and in technology necessitated training beyond the four years of medical school. Furthermore, it was becoming evident that the usual one or two years of internship, consisting of general training, did not provide the specialized skills necessary to improve the quality of care. As scientific and professional leaders in medicine moved toward the establishment of their specialty organizations—the "academies" and "colleges"—the matter of specialty training of residents became of increasing concern, and pressures to alter the pattern of internship training mounted.

Not surprisingly (and as also was the case with interns), hospitals had a large stake in having residents. Residents and interns, "house staff," were a source of cheap labor, and having residency training programs added to an institution's prestige and luster. As a consequence hospitals were pressed to seek approval for specialty training and certification for relatively large numbers of residency positions ("slots"). Each hospital felt that it needed residents, could provide adequate training, and had a stake in expanding the number of available positions. Before long, the total number of residencies far exceeded the number of graduates of American medical schools and bore no relation to actual or projected specialty needs. Yet decertifying residency programs and/or reducing the number of approved residencies a hospital could have was extraordinarily difficult and, had it occurred, would have been extremely painful. The result was that in spite of numerous reports by various commissions, committees, task forces, conferences, and symposia, all of them calling for the rationalization of specialty training, there was no action.

It should be clear, however, that though questions of all kinds were being raised and answers sought, medical education itself was not in turmoil. Indeed, in contrast to the chaotic conditions that prevailed prior to the Flexner Report, by 1940 the pattern of medical education had become stabilized. The trend toward specialization was well under way, and the structure of specialty training programs had become well established. Medical and other health professional organizations grew in numbers and strength. It would have been easy to conclude that all that was needed was a marginal adjustment here and a bit of tweaking there. Such a conclusion would have been valid if medicine and medical education could have stood apart from the society in which they were embedded. But, of course, they could not do so. They necessarily were influenced by the world outside of medicine, and that world, that external environment and its influences, was changing.

Following the end of World War II medical practice incorporated the many recent and newly emerging scientific advances at a rapid pace. The introduction of antibacterial drugs, the growing understanding of the action of hormones, the replacement of blood, plasma, and fluids (procedures that had become common during the war), and the increasing complexity and effectiveness of surgery heightened general expectations for the preservation and lengthening of life. The seemingly infinite productive capacity of the nation during the war, enhanced by the brilliant success of scientists in the application of their knowledge of atomic energy through the Manhattan Project, strengthened the belief in the power of science, technology, and the American economy, and fortified the expectation that any goal could be achieved if sufficient resources were applied to its attainment.

America's medical schools, the major medical research institutions of the country, were receptive to the challenge of unlocking medical secrets and finding cures for various diseases. The long period of institutionalizing the educational program in the prewar years was a time of institutional change, but not of significant institutional growth. But as the nation entered the postwar period of economic advancement, theoretical and methodological advances in the sciences and the ethos of the times stimulated the pressures for research expansion. The universities were attempting to accommodate the influx of veterans (who were assisted in attending college by the G.I. Bill of Rights) and were unable to provide the financial resources required to build the required research infrastructure. The private foundation sector, which had been a major source of support for medical research during the prewar period, found that its resources were inadequate to meet the growing number and size of requests for grants.

It was logical to turn to government for financial help. Support for medical research permitted legislators to assist the health sector without getting involved in politically fractious issues involving medical care delivery, financing, and access. Research appeared to be above the political fray (issues like stem-cell research had not yet entered the public policy arena). Since state budgets were already stretched thin by the rapid growth of state universities and the need to make up for the neglect of capital construction during the depression and the war years, the federal government was called upon to appropriate the necessary funds to underwrite the expansion efforts.

The most suitable locus for a federal research-funding program was the United States Public Health Service, part of the then Federal Security Agency (later to be incorporated into the newly organized Department of Health, Education, and Welfare). The specific subdivision to which appropriations (and through which expenditures) were to be made was the National Institutes of Health (NIH), consisting of a group of individual Institutes that had evolved pragmatically out of concerns with specific organs (for example, the National Heart Institute), diseases (such as the National Cancer Institute), or both (thus the National Institute of Neurological Diseases and Blindness).[11] Although the AMA occasionally expressed its concern about the size of the appropriations and the possible federal control of research, it did not strongly oppose the expansion of NIH support for medical research. It preferred to use its political muscle in vigorous (and successful) opposition to President Truman's legislative proposals in 1948 for national health insurance.

The almost universal acceptance of the importance of funding the medical research effort resulted in its becoming the fastest growing component of all national health expenditures. While total national health expenditures increased from $12.9 billion to $40.7 billion (216 percent) during the 1950–1965 period, research expenditures increased from $117 million to $1.5 billion (1,182 percent) over the same time period. Almost all of the increase was funded by the federal government, whose support for research grew from $79 million (representing 68 percent of all available research dollars) to $1.3 billion (87 percent of all research expenditures) over the same time period.[12]

NIH allocated the federal appropriations to investigators through an innovative scientific-political power structure. In order to assure scientific competence in the awarding of grants (and in order to reduce potential political pressure from legislators who wanted to bring federal dollars to their home districts), the NIH staff created a review process in which each Institute relied on study sections comprised of nongovernmental scientists (drawn mainly from the universities) for initial review of proposals and an advisory council made up of professional persons and citizens-at-large for final ratification. This arrangement enabled a jury system to share the responsibility for scientific judgments while the addition of the advisory council mechanism provided the equivalent of a bicameral process of review. This was important because citizen participation in the council structure provided a defense (though not always sufficient) against the charge that the study section participants were part of an "old boy's network" that had a bias in favor of certain institutions, individuals, and research projects. The elaborate mechanism provided Congress with some assurance that the research dollars it appropriated were being allocated with the advice of the nation's best scientist-citizens.

Nevertheless, it would be incorrect to imply that Congress did not take an active interest in NIH decisions and was fully satisfied with the results of the processes that were based on scientific merit. One continuing bone of contention, in NIH allocations as in many other federal grant programs, related to the concentration of research funds in a relatively limited number of medical schools and universities. On the one hand, no one could easily dispute the proposition that allocations should be based on a proposal's merit. Yet this meant that those schools with a longer tradition of research and a more research-oriented faculty were in a more favorable position to attract additional research grants. Inevitably, representatives from states and congressional districts that did not receive what they perceived as their fair share of the total available dollars protested that they were supporting a system that left their schools further and further behind. NIH had to balance the competing claims for a pure merit system with a "spread the wealth" approach and found that it had to combine both. Even as it allocated research dollars on the basis of scientific merit, it made resources available to help historically less well-endowed schools develop their intellectual capital and research capabilities, thereby enabling them to reach their potential and compete more effectively for future research grants.

The more than tenfold increase in research funds had an important impact on the culture of the medical schools and their parent universities. Since the rapid growth in faculty and physical plant was accomplished mainly by accretion (and expansion of the medical school) rather than by institutional reorganization and the establishment of free-floating institutes, there was a widespread perception that the school's traditional primary mission, teaching medical students, had become diluted. Nor was this mere perception. The "teaching" faculty had relatively fewer resources—fewer dollars for books, supplies, attendance at conferences, and travel—and was often accorded less prestige and status than the "research" faculty because it brought fewer outside dollars into the medical school. Inevitably, there was a relative decline of interest in teaching in favor of research. This phenomenon also occurred in other parts of the modern university and for many institutions continues even today as a major problem needing resolution. Nonetheless, this clash in orientation between research and education first appeared and, perhaps, was more exacerbated in the medical community because of the sheer size and scale of NIH support. This extramural establishment of NIH had a number of important effects on loyalty and decision making in medical education. Many faculty members were much more heavily involved with peer group researchers or with patients than with students. Although a faculty member's loyalties were divided between the granting agency and the university, the greater loyalty tended toward the granting agency, which in many instances was the source of salaries as well as research budgets. Inevitably, many faculty members behaved as if serving on school committees was an intrusion on their time. The school "belonged" to the administration and to those selected faculty members (usually quite senior and well established) who were willing to be involved in school affairs.

The characteristics of what we would term "the sources and uses of funds" had yet another byproduct: they constrained the decision-making power of the dean. An increasing proportion of the total budget came from earmarked or sponsored funds restricted to particular activities. Often these funds were made available to individual grantees with only *pro forma* involvement by the dean's office. The dean had few financial resources that were unencumbered and discretionary and, thus, relatively few ways to move the school in directions that he or she favored or that required priority. Indeed, decisions on funding made in Bethesda, the home of NIH, became instrumental in determining who might be hired and/or promoted—in other words, the makeup of the faculty. As one dean put it at an AAMC institute: "Although the net effect of the relative abundance of such [research] funds has been beneficial, it has, to a rather disquieting extent, taken control of the institution's program and its destiny out of the hand of the university administration and given it to the granting agencies."[13]

The increasing extramural support created a dependence on federal funds undreamt of two decades earlier. As a result some suggested there no longer were private universities and state universities; rather, there were federal and state universities—and the latter had also become very dependent on federal funds. Therefore it was understandable that a tendency to panic developed within the extramural (and university) establishments at suggestions of budget cuts for research or at signs of lagging federal support. That the highest federal officials were aware of the situation was evident in the comment made in 1966 by William D. Carey, Assistant Director of the federal Bureau of the Budget (now the Office of Management and Budget): "Government is not likely to lose sight of the hard reality that in one way or another it will have to provide for the growth and stability of the academic institutions."[14]

The impact of growing research support, need for curriculum revision, and the extension of health services (the three legs of the medical school: research, teaching, and patient care) was an ever-present concern to leaders in medical education and to the organization that represented the medical schools, the AAMC. Such concern was justified and healthy. The numerous conferences and symposia on "current problems in medical education" did not imply that medical leadership was bewailing the various "environmental" changes and doing nothing to adjust to them. Rather, there were ongoing adjustments, and the recognition of and public discussion of issues and problems were paving the way for yet additional needed adjustments. The critical matter is the recognition that medical education, like medical care and research endeavors, necessarily had to be in a continuing state of flux. No issue would be solved; no solution was to hold for all time. In a changing external world with an ever-changing knowledge base, educational issues were being addressed and had to continue to be addressed.

Evidence of this healthy ferment is found in the annual national teaching institutes of the AAMC that had begun in 1953 at the urging of a number of deans.[15] These institutes were each devoted to a different curricular topic and included diverse matters such as physiology, biochemistry, pharmacology, anthropology, appraisal of applicants, ecology of the medical student, medical school administration, medical education, and medical care. These meetings recognized and highlighted the need to accord educational issues high priority in the face of the continuing expansion of research programs. In 1956, in an effort to meet its growing responsibilities more effectively, the AAMC recruited a vigorous, imaginative director, Dr. Ward Darley, the then-president of the University of Colorado. Under his leadership the AAMC began a series of studies on the costs of medical education, which for the first time made specific data available for planning purposes and provided estimates of future needs. Dr. Darley also stimulated research on the characteristics of medical students and the medical schools and made it possible for the Association to render more effective services on student affairs to the medical schools. At various times the AAMC appointed committees of distinguished medical educators to consider the nature of future development in medical education and the role to be played by the Association. These years were not a time when medical educators were asleep or when they behaved as if they believed the sector faced no problems.

Nevertheless, it is important to recognize that even as late as the early 1960s, the AAMC was almost exclusively concerned with issues internal to medical education and to medical schools. The AAMC had not yet fully begun to assert its potential leadership role in speaking for a significant part of American medicine. Neither it nor most medical school deans had developed a capacity to respond to public policy issues in the broader field of medicine and health care. Furthermore, medical school deans faced a full agenda: issues that dealt with school-hospital relations, with town-gown frictions, and with the parent university.

An entirely new set of issues had developed once increasing numbers of private patients with complex medical problems were cared for in university settings. This helped make possible a shift to, and expansion of, a full-time faculty, and that in turn raised inevitable questions concerning the disposition of patient care fees. In earlier times practicing physicians had not viewed the teaching hospital that was taking care of indigent patients as "competition," but that had changed. As hospital physicians cared for an increasing number of patients having health insurance and the ability to pay, many private practitioners (including those with part-time relationships to the medical school and who practiced in the teaching hospital) viewed the school, its hospital, and full-time faculty as direct threats to their practices and opposed the trend.

It was understandable that some deans looked to the AAMC for help on a number of these matters. Nevertheless, extending the AAMC's reach to broader issues had a lower priority. Even so, the leaders of medical education would find that as the AMA became more politically predictable, the AAMC—almost by default—would become more prominent in national health affairs. In the early 1960s that day, however, had not yet come.

In contrast, public health officials as well as legislators were becoming increasingly concerned that, in spite of very considerable research expenditures, the health record of the nation did not exhibit the much hoped-for improvement. This suggested a need for an increased effort to stimulate research and demonstration programs that might have a direct bearing on unresolved health problems. These were the problems that, because they were so common, lacked a high sense of drama, but that (again, because they were so common) were of great importance in determining the health of the population: such matters as infant and maternal mortality, improved immunization rates, nutrition, dental caries, and effects of air pollution. Even as the leadership of NIH and the scientific community spoke about the importance of basic research, those providing the financial support were beginning to ask whether the research accomplishments they heard and read about could be brought out of the laboratory and translated into more effective care and, if that were possible, whether such care would be available to all the people.

This disquietude was not (yet) a threat to the support for research; allocations to science (as applied to medicine) continued to command bipartisan and overwhelming support. Congress annually appropriated more funds than the President requested (although it is true that some Presidents who wanted to submit a low budget did so while counting on Congress to increase it). Nevertheless, the effectiveness and access questions that legislative bodies had begun to ask about medical care indicated a new set of priorities was coming to the fore. Increasingly, issues concerning the distribution of care would command the attention of the taxpayers' representatives.

This concern was part of a dynamic shift in the national perspective. After the depression and World War II, years of turmoil and upheaval, the nation returned President Harry Truman to office. Nevertheless, Congress refused to enact many of the legislative initiatives he proposed. Most conspicuously in the health field, AMA leadership thwarted his efforts to establish a system of national health insurance.[16] When, in 1952, Dwight Eisenhower defeated Adlai Stevenson (as he was to do again in 1956), Americans believed that they had opted for a period of consolidation, perhaps even for tranquility. They surely were incorrect about the latter. During the early 1950s countless individuals and not-for-profit institutions as well as various departments and agencies of government were under siege, as indeed were civil liberties, as Senator Joseph McCarthy led his hunt for communists, fellow-travelers, liberals, and others whom he or his staff aides considered suspect. The early 1950s had another (and more wholesome) stirring: the gathering force of the civil rights movement as a unanimous Supreme Court outlawed racial segregation in education in 1954 and put an end to the legal doctrine that separate could be equal. Yet, if tranquility and normalcy were not to be, the nation did appear to be satisfied with a measure of stability on the legislative front, and there was a general lack of interest in expanding social legislation.

But the period of consolidation was drawing to an end and a restless nation, seemingly ready to embark in new directions, elected John F. Kennedy, a new, young (the first President born in the twentieth century), and vigorous President, in 1960. This was a President who spoke of a "New Frontier" and who had a rich agenda involving numerous international and domestic initiatives. Not least among the latter were issues involving health and medical care, including Medicare, a program to provide hospital insurance to individuals sixty-five years old and over. In no small measure the increase in attention accorded to the financing and distribution of care stemmed from, and was evidence of, the numerous advances made in patient care. The President could not ignore the fact that, in the encounter of patient and physician, there now was more than "a fifty-fifty chance of benefiting from the encounter," but that not everyone had the wherewithal to initiate it.

2 | The Consumer Revolution: Increasing Access to Medical Care

Although physicians were considered authorities on all matters medical, in the mid-twentieth century measures designed to deal with the fact that medical care had become more effective and, not coincidentally, more expensive, did not generally emanate from the medical community. Medical educators were busy educating, medical researchers were busy doing research, medical specialists were consolidating their newly founded societies, and general medical practitioners were represented by the American Medical Association (AMA), which was busy trying to fend off legislative initiatives. As a consequence of the virtual lack of interest in undertaking actions designed to influence events taking place outside the world of medicine, but that nevertheless were affecting medicine in fundamental ways, health care professionals lost control over conditions that would affect their destiny.

The different ways Americans paid for care—matters that were largely decided in the world of politics and commerce—influenced health care priorities, as for example between preventive and acute care, hospital and outpatient care, and primary and specialty care. Thus understanding the development of American health care requires a discussion of health care financing, specifically of health insurance. While the battles over health insurance that took place in the first half of the 1960s are the prelude to the post-1965 story of developments in American medicine, those battles grew out of earlier events.

Early Development of Health Insurance in the United States

The development of health insurance, United States vintage, has a rich history. One place to begin is Dallas, Texas, 1929. While health insurance was not unknown at that time, it was most often found in isolated communities where employers (in railroad and mining, for example) provided insurance to their employees and thereby were able to attract physicians to take care of their workforce. The growth of modern health insurance, however, began in 1929 when an able hospital administrator, Justin Ford Kimball, wanted to make certain that Baylor University Hospital would receive payment for services provided to hospitalized patients. He conceived of the idea of collecting "insurance premiums" in advance and guaranteeing the hospital's services to members of groups subscribing to this arrangement. Further, he found a way to involve employers in the administration of the plan, thus reducing expenses associated with marketing and enrollment. The first such employer was the Dallas school district, which enrolled schoolteachers and collected the biweekly premium of fifty cents.[1] This arrangement—service benefits (so many days in the hospital, and various specified lab tests, rather than dollar payments to the patient after the event) and group enrollment via employer linkage—were to prove critical elements in the expansion of health insurance in the years ahead. Their importance should not be minimized.

During the depression years of the 1930s fewer and fewer patients were admitted to hospitals, for briefer periods of time. An increasing proportion of hospital beds stood empty and an increasing number of bills went unpaid.[2] It should therefore not come as a surprise that what began in Dallas was copied elsewhere. Moreover, the approach was expanded from an arrangement where a group of subscribers was linked to a particular hospital to an arrangement under which the subscriber (and physician) could select any hospital that agreed to be in the plan (and which hospital would dare to be left out?). The orientation to hospital care was not surprising: the hospital was the expensive part of the medical care system, and individual hospitals as well as the American Hospital Association supported such insurance arrangements. Expansion was facilitated through action by the various states, which concluded that because hospitals "guaranteed" the service benefit, hospital association-sponsored not-for-profit plans (which came to be known as "Blue Cross") did not fall under the jurisdiction of insurance commissioners. Because their plans were viewed as "prepayment" rather than insurance, hospitals were not required to post cash reserves to cover their potential liabilities—an important consideration since most hospitals would not have been able to do so.

In return for this (and other) beneficial treatments, the not-for-profit Blue Cross associations in the individual states accepted the responsibility to serve the entire community. While they were not expected to enroll individuals (or groups) who were unable or unwilling to pay the required premium, they were expected to use a "community-rating" standard under which the same premium would be charged to everyone who enrolled, a premium that reflected the average risk in the community and hospital costs associated with that average risk. This meant that whether one was young or old, in a risky and stressful occupation or in a "safe" one, with a healthy lifestyle or without, the premium for the individual or group was not changed to reflect the health experience of the particular subscriber(s) in the previous year. Community-rating was a significant arrangement since, though not designed to achieve universal coverage, it did provide a subsidy to those who were high-risk members of the community. Without that community-rating subsidy, high-risk individuals who were likely to have large medical expenses would have faced prohibitively high premiums.

This arrangement in which lower-risk individuals and groups subsidized others at higher risk, and did so on a voluntary basis, was to prove community-rating's weakness. The voluntary nature of Blue Cross provided for-profit insurers with an opportunity to enter and segment the market by offering premiums based on the health experience of the group with whom they wanted to develop a contractual relationship. If the group were healthier and utilized fewer health care services (as, for example, would be the case if it included few elderly individuals), the experience-rated premium might be considerably less than the community-rated one. Furthermore, the disparity was likely to grow since every time a lower-risk group (in search of a lower premium) opted out of the Blue Cross community-rated arrangement, the average risk for those remaining with the Blues increased and, as a consequence, so did their premium. While the premium differentials were based on risk selection, there surely were employers (and individual subscribers) who ascribed the differences to the presumed efficiency of the commercial for-profit sector, and thereby assuaged whatever guilt they might have felt about "abandoning" the sick and condemning them to higher premiums.

The competitive battle between the not-for-profit Blue Cross Associations that used community-rating and the for-profit commercial insurers who used experience-rating was of fundamental importance. The two approaches represented two philosophies. One relied on cooperation and sharing and was rooted in a view that we are a community, something more than a set of individuals or even of groups. The other limited its cooperation and risk sharing to the members of the group rather than to the greater community. It sought policies that benefited the individual and relied on the individual to search for the maximization of individual well-being. As we shall see, in time the competition forced the Blues to abandon community-rating (or find that their subscribers had abandoned them) and set the stage for the enactment of federal programs to assist the most vulnerable (and therefore most often excluded) members of the community.

Blue Cross was based on hospital service benefits (that is, a guarantee of a set of hospital services). Its "sister" institution, Blue Shield, provided coverage for physician services. Commercial insurers generally provided indemnity benefits (that is, dollar payment after the fact to the subscriber to help meet the cost of the services that had been utilized). In determining the necessary premium, both approaches grounded their calculation on the traditional and familiar fee-for-service payment mechanism. Though fee-for-service was the dominant arrangement, it was not the only type of payment or insurance protection found.

A major alternative to fee-for-service-based insurance protection involved an arrangement under which a prepayment plan agreed to provide all necessary health services (physician as well as hospital, preventive as well as therapeutic) to a group of subscribers for a predetermined monthly premium. In the prepaid group practice (PGP) arrangement, the health plan adopted one of two approaches to obtain the required health care services: either a "staff model" in which it employed salaried physicians or a "group model" in which it contracted for services with a group of physicians for a predetermined sum. The plan's costs depended on the predetermined salary or contractual arrangements with the physicians, rather than (as under fee-for-service insurance arrangements) on the number of services and procedures delivered, billed, and paid for. Its revenues depended on the number of subscribers and the monthly premium charges. Accordingly, the plan budgeted its expenditures within the constraint imposed by the anticipated premium revenues.

Prepaid group practices faced considerable difficulties in establishing themselves and in surviving. Their problems did not lie in the economics of their prepaid arrangements. Rather they lay in the strong opposition of the AMA and its various constituent medical societies, which considered physician contractual or salary relationships violations of the AMA code of ethics. They treated PGP physicians as "black sheep" and denied them membership in the various medical societies and hospital appointments. Therefore, it is understandable that prepaid group practice plans grew relatively slowly (until AMA practices were ruled illegal).

The first PGP plan, sponsored by the Farmers Union and organized in 1929 by Dr. Michael Shadid, a medical practitioner in Elk City, Oklahoma, was subjected to years of harassment by the local and state medical societies. After a suit by the clinic against the medical society for restraint of trade, the society finally settled out of court and admitted the clinic physicians to membership. Nevertheless, this negotiated settlement did not set a legal precedent. That occurred as a consequence of the more prominent conflict involving the Group Health Association prepayment plan in Washington, D.C., which had been organized in 1937. For a period of time its physicians were subjected to pressures that almost drove it out of existence. Suit was brought by the antitrust division of the Department of Justice against the AMA and the Medical Society of the District of Columbia. They were charged with "a conspiracy to hinder and obstruct a group health membership corporation in procuring and retaining on its staff qualified doctors in obtaining access to hospital facilities and to hinder and obstruct its physicians from privilege of consulting with others and using the facilities of hospitals." In January 1943 the Supreme Court of the United States found the AMA guilty of "a conspiracy to restrain trade in the

District of Columbia in violation of the Sherman Anti-Trust Act."[3] It upheld the decision of the United States Court of Appeals for the District of Columbia. That court had stated:

Professions exist because the people believe they will be better served by licensing especially prepared experts to minister to their needs. The licensed monopolies which professions enjoy constitute, in themselves, severe restraints upon competition. But they are restraints which depend upon capacity and training, not special privilege. Neither do they justify concerted criminal action to prevent the people from developing new methods of serving their needs. There is sufficient historical evidence of professional inadequacy to justify occasional popular protests. The better educated laity of today questions the adequacy of present-day medicine. Their challenge finds support, as indicated in the margin, from substantial portions of the medical profession itself. The people give the privilege of professional monopoly and the people may take it away.[4]

The 1943 decision and the spread of employment-linked health insurance in the immediate post–World War II period altered the terrain and ushered in a period of somewhat more rapid PGP growth. This was especially true on the West Coast, where what was to become the largest prepaid group plan had been born out of the efforts of Dr. Sidney Garfield, who had developed a small hospital in the Mojave Desert to serve the needs of the thousands of workers who were building the Los Angeles aqueduct during the Great Depression. He enrolled those workers in a not-for-profit health plan that provided all their medical care for a predetermined amount (ten cents per day for both job and non-job-related medical problems). When the aqueduct project was completed, Henry Kaiser asked Dr. Garfield to replicate his approach for the over 6,000 workers his firm was employing to build the Grand Coulee Dam on the Columbia River in Washington.

Subsequently, during World War II, the Kaiser-Garfield "team" put together a similar plan in Richmond, California, where the Kaiser Shipyards were building Liberty Ships and naval vessels. In 1945, with the conclusion of the war and the rapid drop in employment at the shipyards, the plan's survival appeared problematic. As a consequence it was decided to open the (still) not-for-profit program to the general public in northern California. The organization grew and spread from northern California, first to Los Angeles (with the support of the Longshoremen's and Warehousemen's Union and the Retail Clerks Union) and then beyond the borders of the state.[5] At about the same time, in 1947, the then-mayor of New York City, Fiorello LaGuardia, and the New York municipal labor unions founded the Health Insurance Plan of New York (HIP), an important East Coast addition to the prepaid group practice "movement." As we shall see, these various PGPs, but especially the Kaiser Plan, played an important role in the development of the health maintenance organization initiative under President Nixon.

The 1940s: The Advantages of Group Enrollment

In the postwar period other industrial nations adopted national plans designed to achieve universal coverage (for all medical care, as in the British National Health Service, or, initially, for hospital care, as in Canadian Medicare). The United States instead opted for voluntary employment-related health insurance and used public policy to encourage its further development. The critical aspects assisting the growth and expansion of voluntary health insurance (whether fee-for-service or prepaid group practice) in the United States were group enrollment, employment linkage, and favorable tax treatment.

Group enrollment meant a reduction in a wide variety of administrative expenses, for example those associated with marketing and collecting premiums in bulk rather than from individuals. Group enrollment also meant that the power of numbers could be mobilized on behalf of the subscribers. The insurer did not have to worry about self-selection aspects that might induce sicker individuals to join and healthier ones to opt out. Instead, the average risk for the group (and under community-rating, for the community) applied to all. This was what Winston Churchill had termed "bringing the magic of averages to the rescue of millions."[6] If the group were large enough, no catastrophic event, however costly, would have a significant impact on the premium. In turn this reduced the possibility of discrimination by the group's sponsor (most often the employer) against individuals who for whatever reason were higher risk. Of course, the corollary was that small groups were vulnerable to such untoward events. With the exception of community-rating, it was difficult for small firms with few employees to purchase the requisite insurance since insurers charged additional amounts to protect themselves against these low-probability, but very expensive, events.

It is important to recognize that the lower premiums associated with group arrangements did not benefit individuals who, for whatever reason, were not members of any group purchase or enrollment program. Building on the experience in Dr. Kimball's plan for Dallas schoolteachers, most groups were organized around employment. Thus individuals who were not employed (including retirees) or who were employed by an employer who did not help sponsor a plan were usually excluded from group coverage.

Because the most common group arrangement and linkage involved employment, this pattern had many administrative and enrollment advantages, especially so during the Second World War when America bounced back from the depths of the depression. Between 1939 and 1944 the unemployment rate dropped from 17.2 percent to 1.2 percent, and the Gross National Product grew by almost 75 percent in real (corrected for inflation) terms. In an effort to control inflationary pressures on the prices for consumer goods in short supply and on wages in a full-employment economy, the federal government instituted price and wage controls. Nevertheless, it did permit additions (within limits) to fringe benefits, including health insurance. Given the high levels of taxation on wartime increases in profits, employers were willing to augment their contribution for health care coverage (or to offer such coverage if they had not previously done so). The costs of insurance, after all, were being paid by dollars that in large measure would otherwise have been paid in taxes.

And there was more: the amount that the employer paid for health insurance was considered a "cost of doing business." It was a cost, akin to wages and other items that were legitimate expenses and deductions from what otherwise would have been profits. Yet at the same time the value to the individual of the premium dollars paid on his or her behalf was not considered as income on which the worker would have to pay income and (perhaps) Social Security taxes. The consequent decrease in government revenues provided a substantial subsidy toward the purchase of health insurance. It should be pointed out that the failure to tax the value of the premiums as income meant that the subsidy was greater and worth more the higher the individual's income and the greater the individual's marginal tax rate. The CEO received a larger tax benefit subsidy than did the secretary.

This tax provision was maintained as part of the tax code in the postwar period. Given the tax advantages and a National Labor Relations Board ruling that an employer who refused to bargain over health insurance coverage was engaging in an unfair labor practice, health insurance benefits quickly became part of normal collective bargaining. Unions (and their members) understood that, because of taxes, a dollar in pretax wages would become less than a dollar in take-home pay and, therefore, could purchase less than a dollar's worth of health insurance. Conversely, an employer contribution of a dollar toward health insurance premiums would purchase a full dollar's worth of coverage. It is not surprising that unions wanted to increase the employer contribution toward health insurance (even at the expense of wages) and that this tax benefit helped fuel the rapid growth of insurance.

At the entry of the United States into the war at the beginning of 1942, Blue Cross covered 6 million subscribers; by 1946 enrollment had exploded to 18.9 million. Commercial insurance covered some 3.7 million persons in 1941 and 10.5 million by 1946. Further rapid growth followed: from a 1946 total of 32 million persons covered by Blue Cross, commercial plans, PGPs, and independent plans, to 53 million in 1948, and to 77 million by 1951.[7] As a consequence of changing patterns of medical care, in particular in the utilization of hospital services, much of this increase in coverage was for hospital care, creating a not-so-subtle perverse incentive to hospitalize individuals. This was the case even for diagnostic tests that could have been performed on a less costly outpatient basis. Over time the hospital thus became all the more important and central to the delivery of health care services, a phenomenon not unrelated to the expansion in the number of hospitals and of beds following the 1946 enactment of the Hospital Survey and Construction Act (the Hill-Burton Act). In a reciprocal manner, since medical care became more costly, insurance became more useful (indeed, necessary). In turn, the presence of insurance helped underwrite a buildup of resources and an upgrading of technology that added to costs and made insurance even more valuable.

The 1950s: The Dynamics of Being "Left Out"

It can be said that insurance made health sector expansion possible; it can also be said that health sector expansion helped generate the increase in insurance. America was entering a period of extraordinarily rapid growth of its health sector. As a result of the expansion and of the rise in costs of and expenditures for medical care, it was also entering a period of stress on existing arrangements. Perhaps the most important pressure on the system came from the mounting difficulty that Blue Cross faced in attempting to maintain its commitment to consumer-rating. The Blues began to shift to a system of "adjusted" or "modified" community-rating that took account of gender and age in setting premiums and, when this proved competitively insufficient, to a system incorporating experience-rating. This of course had adverse implications for higher-risk groups and individuals who had been beneficiaries of the previously available subsidy.

Nevertheless, private health insurance continued to grow so rapidly that many persons believed that further expansion of the Blues, commercial carriers, and PGPs and independents would enable the United States to reach universal coverage. They agreed that perhaps some limited government programs might be needed to assist low-income population groups, but surely it was not necessary to contemplate enactment of a Truman-like comprehensive national government plan. As the nation entered the 1950s it was easy to ignore the numerous recommendations of President Truman's Commission on the Health Needs of the Nation. Attitudes toward the health sector were not at variance with the view that the Eisenhower victory was a mandate to consolidate and expand trends already under way, not to embark on new and bold initiatives.

Yet the very expansion (but nonuniversal nature) of private employment-linked health insurance increased the pressures on those who did not have insurance, but received their medical care from a health care system that was increasingly costly (in no small measure because of the insurance that others used and that financed health sector expansion). These "left out" persons were not linked to employer-provided (and subsidized) health insurance. Many were retired or had no relationship to the labor market. Many others were full-time workers, but at wages so low that it was unreasonable to argue that they would have been better off substituting health insurance for some of their already inadequate wage income. Some were self-employed and faced the insurance market as individuals (subject to higher premiums because of self-selection) rather than as members of a group. Nor could it escape notice that the "haves" and "have-nots" were distributed very unequally by race: the probability that a person of color would not have health insurance was much higher than was the case for the rest of the population. Increasingly those who were left out and left behind had to turn to private charity or, if available, the county or city public hospital. And increasingly the hospital emergency room was their main source of care, a phenomenon that inflated the costs of medical care and left the crowded and overworked emergency room less able to handle true emergencies.

The impact of these various developments was made more acute by the scientific revolution and the resultant advances in medicine. In a much earlier time, when medicine could do much less for patients, being "left out" was not as consequential. That was no longer true. As the renowned medical historian Richard H. Shryock had written:

Hence there gradually evolved in educated minds, a syllogism of some such form as this: Medical science can now prevent or cure certain major diseases. Many people continue to suffer from these very diseases. Ergo, medical science does not serve the people as it should. The most obvious explanation was to be found in the mounting costs of service. Here, again, it is to be noted that it was the very progress which physicians had made in science, which involved them in new difficulties in the practice of their art. Technical improvements led to simultaneous increase in the demand for medical services and in the price that must be paid for them. And so the more that people trusted medical aid, the less they could afford it. Here was a serious and unexpected impasse in the public relations of the profession.[8]

Medicine could do more and, because it seemed inevitable that it would continue to advance, having access to care was ever more important. Moreover, one could sensibly argue that since the private competitive sector appeared unable to achieve a goal of reasonable distributional equity in access to insurance and medical care, there was an increasing need for government intervention.

It would not be until the mid-1960s that the nation would resolve the debate about the way to assist the aged, one of the groups without insurance, and choose between a federal social insurance program for all the aged and a welfare-oriented, means-tested, state-administered assistance program for low-income elderly. The debate, however, began in the latter 1950s, at the beginning of Eisenhower's second term when Congressman Aimee Forand of Rhode Island introduced a social insurance bill providing for hospital insurance for Social Security beneficiaries, financed through an increase in the Social Security payroll tax.

Why focus on the elderly? It, of course, was true that elderly Social Security beneficiaries were finding it increasingly difficult to obtain affordable health insurance. They were not members of an insurance group and did not have a link to employment or an employer subsidy for the purchase of a medical care policy. That, however, was equally true of many others. Various factors did set the elderly apart and made it easier to conceive of a program that would provide them with a hospital insurance policy. Because of the influence of age, they were more likely to need and to utilize health services. In 1963, for example, the elderly accounted for 9.4 percent of the population, but 19.7 percent of total medical care spending.[9] Furthermore, unlike other individuals whose socioeconomic and demographic characteristics might change —for example, today's uninsured might have insurance in some future period and today's low-income individual might have higher income tomorrow—the aged were a more stable group. Once one was a

Social Security beneficiary (retired and age sixty-five or over) one would not become younger in some future period. Thus there was no need for periodic checking of eligibility.

Additionally, if one were arguing for a social insurance approach, it made sense (and was administratively efficient) to begin with a group that was already in the social insurance system, already eligible for and receiving Social Security benefits. Finally, the aged, though defined as individuals for insurance enrollment purposes, were a highly visible, vocal, and active group in the world of politics, one that exhibited above-average political participation and voting behavior.

The story of the period from 1957 when, in limited form, what came to be known as "Medicare" was first proposed, till 1965 when a far more comprehensive Medicare program was enacted, has an underlying story line: an eight-year debate about the mechanism the federal government should use in helping increase access to medical care. At a deeper level, this was a debate about the proper role for the federal government and the individual states, about the choice between a focus on the individual or on the group, and the appropriate definition of the "group." This, of course, was not a new debate, nor was it a debate that would be resolved for all time. In 1965 it was resolved in relation to Medicare, but the debate continues about other programs and, as we shall see, still continues even around Medicare.

The 1960s: Presidential Involvement and the Bumper Crop of Health Legislation

While the debate about medical care insurance for the aged was, as noted, the underlying (and divisive) motif for the eight years that encompassed the last years of Eisenhower's presidency, the almost three years of Kennedy's, and the first years of Johnson's, this was not the only measure on the congressional health agenda (or on the agendas of the various state legislatures). During those years various programs designed to address, perhaps some believed even "solve," various troubling health and health care issues were adopted. In largest measure they focused on the resource and supply side of the medical care equation rather than, as with insurance, on demand. Not unexpectedly, they reflected the interests of the President and of key legislators and the knowledge, perspectives, and influence of medical scientists, including the leadership of the National Institutes of Health. During the Kennedy years, for example, the President's personal concern about the problems of mental retardation—an affliction of one of his sisters—led to the formation of a distinguished panel of experts and nonprofessionals that resulted in a set of recommendations to Congress and the enactment of the Mental Retardation Facilities Construction Act of 1963, designed to increase and improve clinical facilities for treatment.[10] Similarly, when the Joint Commission on Mental Illness and Health (formed during the Eisenhower administration and encompassing a wide variety of groups and constituencies) issued its final report in 1961,[11] the administration proposed and Congress enacted the Community Mental Health Centers Act of 1963. The Act recognized the need to deal with the deterioration of state mental hospitals and the construction and operation of community mental health centers. It enabled the provision of services to patients who, as a consequence of the development of more effective psychotropic drugs, were being discharged from the large state facilities.

Other potential initiatives (beyond Presidential support for Medicare) were being readied for inclusion in the Kennedy administration's health agenda for 1964, the run-up to the election, and subsequently for the (presumed) second term during which the President expected to have a strengthened congressional majority. None of this was to be, because of what happened in November of 1963 in Dallas. It fell to the new President, Lyndon Baines Johnson, to build upon Kennedy's agenda and to develop his own set of health initiatives.

Early in 1964 in a message to Congress the President announced the formation of a Commission on Heart Disease, Cancer, and Stroke—espousing the "killer-diseases" concept that had been passed on from the previous administration. The Commission was appointed in March 1964 and submitted its report in December of the same year, a timetable that provided further evidence, if any were needed, that this President would be extraordinarily active in pursuit of legislative accomplishments. The Commission made numerous recommendations, three of which formed the basis for proposals to the House and Senate.

As often occurs, Congress modified the objectives and the proposals before enacting, in 1965, the legislation that would provide support for the planning and establishment of a set of Regional Medical Programs (RMP) for research, training, and continuing education in the fields of heart disease, cancer, stroke, and related diseases. Congress was explicit in stating that the various ends of improving the knowledge base and the training and education of practitioners, and thereby making possible the latest advances in diagnosis and treatment, were to be accomplished without interfering in any way with the patterns or methods of financing of patient care, professional practice, or the administration of any existing institutions.

This explicit "noninterference" provision reflected the concerns of the AMA, the American Hospital Association, and a number of voluntary organizations such as the American Heart Association and the American Cancer Society, all of which wanted assurance that prevailing patterns and relationships (including, of course, financial relationships) between patients and practitioners would not be disturbed.[12] In spite of the President's desires—and this was a President who was a master legislative strategist and tactician—Congress demonstrated, as it had so often done, that it was much more amenable to increasing funds for research and training than to undertaking actions that might impinge on or alter prevailing access to services arrangements.

Yet this was a President whose larger visions were not to be denied. The enactment of the Civil Rights Act of 1964 (after a long filibuster) and of the Elementary and Secondary Education Act in 1965 (after years of attempts and failures) were better guides to what he might (and would) accomplish than the failure to get all he wanted in the legislation on heart disease, cancer, and stroke. President Johnson elevated the previous administration's concern about poverty into a "War on Poverty," and in order to attack poverty in a comprehensive manner presided over the enactment of the Economic Opportunity Act, which, among other things, set up the Office of Economic Opportunity (OEO) under the Executive Office of the President to develop and administer a wide variety of antipoverty programs. The tragedy of Vietnam had not yet significantly intruded upon his plans for "The Great Society."

Even as he was laying the groundwork for yet another attempt to enact Medicare, Johnson was urging rapid implementation of programs developed by OEO to assist the poor in achieving access to health services. Among these programs two stand out, not only because they were bold and imaginative, and not only because they accomplished much that was useful and that helped many children and adults who needed help, but also because they and/or their activities still remain in place four decades later. The first is Head Start, which began in 1965 and moved with extraordinary speed from a planning mode to a program that provided education, health, and welfare services for almost 600,000 children, job opportunities for parents, and nonpartisan political involvement under the aegis of community participation for many neighborhood residents. While the ongoing program was about preparing children for school (to give them a "Head Start"), it would be incorrect to assume (as many did) that meant attention was paid solely to educational matters. Education and preparation for a good education could not occur on an empty stomach or under the stress of illness. Thus Head Start included health assessments and appropriate health care. The value and the contribution of the program are demonstrated by Head Start's survival today. In no small measure this is the result of the support it receives at the community level from parents, teachers, and concerned citizens who see, understand, and value its accomplishments.

OEO also created an important additional intervention that dealt with health care: the neighborhood health center program.[13] Those who are familiar with today's community health centers (many of whose beginnings lie in this program) may fail to appreciate that in the mid-sixties this contribution to the health system's infrastructure was both novel and imaginative. These centers, often collaborating with medical schools, health departments, professional societies, or local antipoverty agencies, provided family-centered comprehensive care. By doing so in an institutional framework, they offered a measure of economic security to physicians (making it possible to redistribute physician resources), trained and utilized appropriate nonprofessional personnel in promoting health education and health care, provided employment as health workers (and the necessary training and on-the-job experience) to neighborhood residents, and in doing that and more helped build community institutions in what so often were fragmented neighborhoods. The wonder, perhaps, is not that the centers were successful; the wonder is that so much that was learned and that had wide applicability concerning the redistribution of resources and the delivery of health care to the greater society has been largely ignored.

Important as these (and other efforts) were in increasing the services available to the poor, there was little question that the Johnson administration's efforts and accomplishments in the health arena would be judged by its record on Medicare. The years of effort to enact a social insurance system for financing hospital insurance for the aged meant that Medicare had symbolic importance that extended beyond its protection of millions of senior citizens against the economic impact of illness.[14] Moreover, many supporters viewed Medicare, even despite its absence of coverage for physicians' services, as a "building block," as the cornerstone of a program that, in due course, would be expanded and cover all the population. If this first step failed to be enacted (or were to fail to be successfully implemented), hope for a more comprehensive and inclusive universal program would necessarily be shelved.

The reader who knows today's Medicare program may wonder why we refer to the Medicare hospital insurance program when, in fact, Medicare has (and from enactment has had) a Part A that primarily provides hospital insurance and a Part B that in largest measure addresses itself to physician services. The answer lies in the fact that from the beginning of the debate proponents hoped that by limiting themselves to hospital care they would minimize AMA opposition and also reduce program costs and thus the need for an even larger Social Security tax. Advocates modeled the program after Blue Cross and spoke about putting the equivalent of the well-known Blue Cross card into the wallets and pocketbooks of elderly Americans.

In 1960, in the prelude to the Kennedy-Nixon election, opposition to the social insurance program came not from those who thought the hospital program incomplete and inadequate, but from critics led by Senator Robert Taft, a powerful conservative Ohio Republican. They supported a program that would provide financial assistance to states that desired to participate in the program. The combination of federal and state funds and premiums from eligible individuals (presumably) would help very low income individuals purchase a health insurance policy that covered hospital and physician services. But the proposal required that the individual meet a significant deductible before receiving any reimbursed benefits and pay a percentage of the approved costs incurred after the deductible was reached. Thus, though providing more comprehensive benefits than the original hospital-only approach, the Taft alternative would have been available solely to those relatively few individuals who resided in a participating state, met the extremely low income limit, and nevertheless were able to meet the required premium, deductible, and co-insurance outlays.

This and the social insurance approach vied for support during the 1960 Kennedy-Nixon Presidential campaign debates. The members of the large and solid bloc of southern Democrats were caught between their conservative views (but aware that the "welfare" approach supported by Republicans would not help their low-income constituents or low-income states) and the social insurance program that they rejected out of principle. They developed a third approach: an expansion of the existing 1950 program that provided help to the states to pay for medical care for those aged who were so poor that they were receiving cash assistance under the federal old-age assistance program. Under the new proposal eligibility would be expanded and would no longer depend on the receipt of cash assistance. Low-income status would suffice and the number receiving medical assistance would rise. In many respects the proposal was similar to that promoted by Senator Taft. It was more generous, but its real strength (at least for the southern members of Congress) was that it was "theirs."

This measure, the Kerr-Mills approach (named after two Democratic sponsors, Senator Robert Kerr of Oklahoma and Representative Wilbur Mills of Arkansas, the powerful chairman of the House Ways and Means Committee), though rejected by both Presidential candidates, was enacted with overwhelming support by the southern bloc. Yet it was evident that the issue had not been resolved by this hardly adequate compromise. Given that President Kennedy was committed to the social insurance alternative, the issue stayed alive through his administration. Nevertheless, the split in the Democratic ranks between southern conservatives (who had not left the Democratic Party to become Republicans) and northern liberals made it impossible to move the President's proposals forward. In 1962 the President's program was defeated by a vote of 52 to 48. Though Democrats controlled the Senate by a margin of 64 to 36 members, 21 Democrats (largely from the South) deserted the President while only 5 Republicans crossed the aisle to vote with the majority of Democrats.

In November 1963 the mantle of leadership passed to President Johnson, who creatively managed to link an increase in Social Security benefits to enactment of Medicare and then, in order to keep Medicare alive after the legislation failed to pass, managed to convince the Senate not to grant the benefit increase, but to return to the linked issue after the 1964 election. That election was to prove decisive: Johnson defeated Barry Goldwater overwhelmingly; the Democrats captured both House and Senate by more than a two-to-one majority and increased their strength in the North where pro-Medicare members defeated Republican opponents. It did not take long for the body politic (and for Congressman Mills who chaired the committee that would consider Medicare) to recognize that the long battle about Medicare was drawing to a close.

Yet there was to be a stunning unanticipated event. The American Medical Association mounted a last-ditch effort to derail the legislation and proposed its own "Eldercare" proposal to provide both hospital and physician coverage, but through the states and only to those individuals who were "truly" needy (an initiative not unlike the existing Kerr-Mills program, but more expansive). The AMA spent over a million dollars emphasizing that its proposal covered physician services and was far more comprehensive than the "inadequate" administration proposal sponsored by Senator Clinton Anderson of New Mexico and Representative Cecil King of California. Furthermore, it pointed out that the administration's program was "inadequate" on yet another score: it would not address the plight of those in poverty who were not aged. While not offering a way to meet that problem, the

AMA could claim that the administration program was being "oversold" on both counts.

The administration, even under Kennedy, had already feared the negative public reaction when the public discovered that by excluding physician services Medicare provided far less comprehensive benefits than potential beneficiaries expected. Now it responded to the effectiveness of the AMA campaign in two important and surprising ways. It grafted a Medicare Part B physicians' services voluntary program (paid for in part out of general revenues and in part by the enrollee) onto the Medicare hospital program. It also supported (and Congress enacted) a new program, Medicaid (Title 19 of the Social Security Act), that would pay for medical care services and nursing-home long-term care for low-income individuals (of all ages) who were receiving cash-assistance welfare payments (poor blind, or aged, or disabled persons, members of families eligible for Aid to Families with Dependent Children, and certain categories of pregnant women). In addition, in an extraordinarily complex set of eligibility and funding criteria, the states could cover and the federal government would share in the costs of care for additional individuals.

Thus, as a result of a landslide election, as a memorial to the assassinated President, under the guidance of a President with legendary legislative skills and of a chairman of the House Ways and Means Committee whose influence in shepherding the bill was immense, and aided by the miscalculation by the AMA, a far more comprehensive measure than was originally proposed by Congressman Forand was enacted. It covered three million additional aged persons who were not part of the Social Security system, allowed more days of hospital and nursing-home care, created a voluntary (but heavily subsidized) program to cover out-of-hospital services, and, though separately enacted, provided Medicaid assistance for acute and long-term care to many of the nation's poor. Medicare (Title 18 of the Social Security Act) was signed into law in Independence, Missouri, in the presence of Harry Truman, on July 30, 1965. The law was to be implemented on July 1, 1966, less than a year later. This was to be a formidable undertaking.

The Medicare program has changed over the forty years since its enactment. Because of inflation that, of course, is true of the deductibles, the premiums under Part B, the Medicare-approved fees to physicians, and the level of reimbursements to hospitals. In addition, as we shall see, there have been changes in the method of reimbursing hospitals and in the assistance to teaching hospitals for educational and training costs. There have been adjustments as well that attempt to reflect and adapt to new patterns in the organization of care (such as HMOs and hospices) and new benefits (such as pharmaceuticals).

Yet many aspects of the basic structure of Medicare remain in place. The beneficiary is entitled to sixty days of semiprivate hospital care (after paying a large basic deductible), another thirty days of care with a daily payment of one-quarter of the deductible, and a lifetime "reserve" of sixty days (at one-half of the deductible per day). A benefit period begins with the first day in hospital and ends when the patient has been out of hospital for sixty consecutive days; the beneficiary may have an unlimited number of benefit periods. Under Part A there are additional provisions (and limitations) that apply to skilled nursing or rehabilitation services as well as home health, psychiatric hospital, and hospice services. Under the voluntary Part B (the premium is typically simply deducted from the Social Security benefit check) the enrollee receives assistance in paying for physicians' services, various outpatient, home health, and other nonroutine services, and durable equipment and supplies, such as wheelchairs and pacemakers. The beneficiary pays an annual deductible and, after the deductible, 20 percent of the Medicare-approved charge (which may be less than the actual charge).[15] It is easy to understand why many individuals who have the financial resources to do so purchase a Medicare Supplement policy that covers the deductibles and co-insurance costs.

It is important to note that Medicare was structured in what may appear a complex manner, because it followed patterns already in place in the private insurance market. Medicare did not attempt to alter traditional health care arrangements. Indeed, Medicare was specifically enjoined (in much the same way as in the heart, cancer, and stroke legislation) from any such interference. The House Ways and Means Committee put it quite directly when it stated: "The bill specifically prohibits the Federal Government from exercising supervision or control over the practice of medicine, the manner in which medical services are provided, and the administration or operation of medical facilities."[16]

One wonders whether members of Congress really believed that federally funded Medicare and Medicaid with a state-federal financing structure under which states paid bills on behalf of Medicaid recipients (note the difference between a social insurance and welfare orientation: the one speaks of "beneficiaries," the other of "recipients") would serve as mere conduits for billions of dollars without affecting the medical care system. One wonders whether they really believed that with the enactment of Medicare and Medicaid they had done so much to solve medical care problems that they would not have to deal with a health care agenda for some considerable time. If there were members who so believed, they were to be disappointed. Not only would Medicare and Medicaid (and the dollars they spent and the ways they spent them) raise new sets of issues and new priorities, not only would their structures affect and distort the structure of the delivery system and exacerbate health care inflation, not only would there still be large numbers of individuals and families without health care insurance, but all these (and more) would be further affected by the dynamic and ever-changing nature of our society. Even as Medicare and Medicaid were signed into law, our Vietnam commitments were expanding and America was entering a period of great flux. Could one imagine that health care would be exempt from change, that health care would be an island of stability in an ocean of turmoil?

Part II

IN THE WAKE OF MEDICARE
AND MEDICAID (1965–1985)

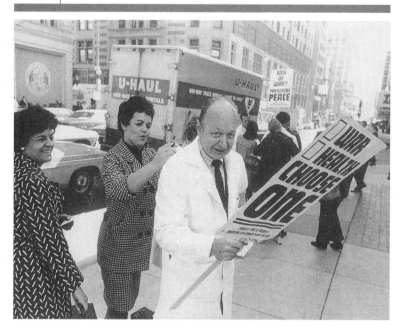

Dean Robert H. Ebert of Harvard Medical School lends his back for the signing of a petition protesting the Vietnam War on Moratorium Day (October 15, 1969) in downtown Boston. Photograph from the Harvard Medical Library in the Francis A. Countway Library of Medicine.

3 | Emerging Tensions between Regulation and Market Forces: Dealing with Growth

Many Americans may find it difficult to appreciate the impact of the social ferment of the mid-1960s associated with the civil rights revolution and President Lyndon Johnson's declaration of a "War on Poverty." The 2000 census reports that today's median age is 35.3 years. Thus over half our population had not yet been born four decades ago when the Civil Rights Act of 1964 was enacted and when the President articulated his goal of creating a "Great Society." They may not understand the significance of the Voting Rights Act of 1965, of place names like Montgomery or Selma, of terms such as "Freedom Riders" and "Freedom Summer." They may not realize that the term "Great Society" was not used as a mere rhetorical flourish, but that it defined and embodied a legislative program and called for a national commitment. The attempt to attain that goal, which included actions on civil rights, necessarily affected every part of American society. The ways that health care services were financed and delivered as well as the ways that health professionals were educated and trained were not immune to the surrounding ferment.

Social Ferment and the Medical Schools

As part of the larger society, medicine was called on to increase access to and improve the quality of health care services and thus help meet the health needs of the poor and members of minority groups. Medical education and medical educators were expected to contribute to the attainment of those goals. It was also anticipated that they would pursue policies designed to foster the diversity of students in the health professions.

One of us, Rashi Fein, recalls that at a meeting of President Johnson's health task force prior to the 1964 election, the President asked that the group prepare a document outlining the health legislation that would make America a better and healthier nation "twenty-five years from now." He specifically cautioned against a focus on the present and the immediate future and told the panel members to dare to dream and to "think big" and that since he, not we, had the political know-how, we were to tell him what was needed, not what we believed could be enacted. The political will to accomplish these various purposes was manifested in the bumper crop of health legislation enacted in 1965.[1] We do not use that term lightly. Much more legislation was enacted and many more programs were expanded than the task force dared to outline—the President's definition of "big" exceeded ours: community mental health centers, Office of Economic Opportunity neighborhood health centers, Head Start, children and youth projects, regional medical programs, comprehensive health planning, multicounty demonstration health facilities, public health formula grants, project grants for health service demonstrations, the Nurses Training Act, the Allied Health Professions Training Act, support of medical, dental, optometry, pharmacy, and veterinary education, and Medicare and Medicaid. Supported by tens of millions of Americans and backed by numerous and comprehensive legislative initiatives, the goals of President Johnson's "Great Society" appeared attainable.

Yet, even as the various programs to expand and redistribute resources, services, and access to them—as well as educational and training opportunities—were being implemented, other social and political forces began to displace the national commitment to the civil rights revolution and the War on Poverty. The expanding war in Vietnam became the focus of the President's attention and consumed the human and financial resources required to sustain his social agenda and the programs it encompassed. Thus, in spite of the success of antipoverty programs such as Head Start and community/neighborhood health centers, the momentum for expanding these and other efforts was lost. Not only was there the inevitable diversion of money from social programs located in the various departments and agencies of government and in the Office of Economic Opportunity (OEO), which housed and coordinated federal antipoverty efforts, but much of the energy and effort that focused on and supported the war on poverty was diverted into protests against the war in Vietnam.

These protests were pervasive and touched every facet of American life. Inevitably, they had a very substantial impact within the universities and their various faculties. While the protest movement was most evident among undergraduates on college and university campuses, medical schools were not insulated, especially since many of their students had been involved in the movement during their earlier college student days. Many medical school faculty members, dismayed that the protests might interfere with training requirements and activities, called upon the students to "behave," as if their role as citizens was secondary to their role as students. Nevertheless, as is well known, the protests continued and gathered force. As an example, in the spring of 1969, Harvard medical students, joining with students in other parts of the university, refused to attend classes and (after a vote) quite literally went out on strike. Some members of the faculty supported the students; others argued that such actions were "irresponsible." In fact, however, striking students formed their own study groups and informal tutorials, continued to prepare to become physicians, and understood the contribution that residency training would make in equipping them for the world of practice.

The students were not alone in mounting protests. On October 15, 1969, as part of the nationwide Vietnam War Moratorium, Dr. Robert H. Ebert, the dean of the Harvard Medical School, together with the heads of a number of Harvard's teaching hospitals, all dressed in white coats on which their names were visibly displayed, went to downtown Boston to gather signatures on petitions and close to 100,000 postcards against the war. The *Boston Globe* reported that over six hundred Boston physicians, medical personnel, and students were involved in the street corner postcard campaign or in hospital-based teach-ins.[2] Nor was Harvard unique: similar protests were taking place in colleges and universities across the nation.

Medical schools were a part of, not apart from, the world outside the classroom, laboratory, and hospital walls. Thus it is not surprising that along with the newfound political activism, there were changes in student behavior. Past norms of personal dress and demeanor no longer prevailed.[3] Students wanted, and often were given, much more participation in the governance of the medical schools.[4] Throughout society old patterns that were familiar and stable were being questioned. Bob Dylan provided the correct description: "The times they are a-changin'."

In a number of schools students expressed what could be interpreted as an antiacademic orientation. Focusing on "the immediate," this often took the form of denigrating faculty involvement in research and advocating more emphasis on services for the poor. An anecdote is illustrative. While one of us (Julius Richmond) was serving as dean of the medical school of the State University of New York at Syracuse, he was presented with a student demand that faculty members give up research time in order to expand clinical services to the poor. The dean reminded the students that a graduate of the school, Dr. Paul Parkman, had developed a method for culturing rubella virus, thus making possible the development of a vaccine. He suggested that Dr. Parkman would prevent more deaths and disability by working in his laboratory than any medical school class would eliminate by delivering needed health care services even over the lifetimes of all its members.[5] The dean made clear that there was a need for "balance."

The sixties were a chaotic period in medical schools and for medical education. Nevertheless, as was also true for the larger society, it was a period that, though characterized by turmoil, brought enduring benefits. Especially evident was the new emphasis on greater diversity in the student body and, though slow-paced, in the faculty (in gender, race, ethnicity, and economic background). The face of medicine was becoming more reflective of the face of America. Furthermore, there was a legacy of important health legislation that expanded access to medical care services: most especially Medicare, and, though structured quite differently, Medicaid.

Rising Expenditures

The late sixties and early seventies were years characterized by rapid inflation, especially in health care.[6] Prices and expenditures for medical care increased at rates not previously seen. President Richard Nixon, confronted with "stagflation" (that is, a stagnant economy and declining stock market combined with inflation and a rising Consumer Price Index) unexpectedly (and especially so for a Republican president) implemented a set of price controls, effective on August 15, 1971. These controls provided a respite in the health arena: over the next year the Consumer Price Index for medical care service rose by only 2.5 percent. Nevertheless, after the controls were relaxed and then lifted, there again was an extremely rapid increase in health care prices and expenditures.

While the Consumer Price Index for medical care services increased by 3.7 percent in calendar year 1972 and 4.4 percent in 1973, it rose a full 10.3 percent in 1974.[7] (See Figure 1.) It became clear that the surge in medical care prices and the accompanying rapid growth in personal health care expenditures were creating severe problems for individuals who faced rising insurance premiums (often at the expense of potential wage increases); for private sector employers who contributed in full or in part to employee health insurance; and for all levels of government. A decade earlier, in the early 1960s, the issue of coverage and expansion of access (especially for retirees) commanded public attention. Now, in the early 1970s, a response to rising prices and expenditures was required. The issue of access was replaced by a newfound emphasis on finding ways to moderate the cost increases, that is, on cost containment.

It is useful to note the different meanings of the term "health care costs." Sometimes it is used to refer to an increase in prices; at other times it refers to an increase in expenditures. Though the former contributes to the latter, there is a substantial difference between the two concepts. The increase in expenditures may reflect a change in prices for various medical services (often termed "costs" of care), but may be due as well to population growth (especially in age groups that utilize more medical care), an expansion in quantity and intensity of services (including newly developed interventions), a greater use of technology, and, occasionally, costly quality enhancements. It can be argued that increases in expenditures are associated with economic affluence, that is, that we value health care and that a richer society will be able

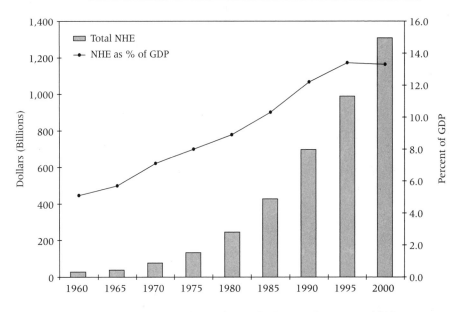

Figure 1. National Health Expenditures, Current Dollars and Percentage of GDP, 1960–2000. *Source:* Data for 1960–1990 from National Center for Health Statistics, *Health, United States, 1998* (Washington, D.C., 1998), Table 115; data for 1995 and 2000 from National Center for Health Statistics, *Health, United States, 2003* (Washington, D.C., 2003), Table 112.

to, and will choose to, spend more on health care of all kinds. It can also be argued that an increase in a nation's expenditures for health may be associated with improvements in the health status of the population (although this is not necessarily the case across countries).[8] Thus increases in expenditures that reflect increases in the utilization of services, efforts in research, and infrastructure expansion are not necessarily undesirable. Nevertheless, expenditure increases do place a burden on the various payers, and it is evident that these rapid increases can be slowed if prices for medical services can be stabilized.

Initially, federal and state authorities as well as private insurers turned to regulation and to attempts to set and control prices and utilization. Special efforts involved such matters as "prior approval" and "second opinion." Hikes in Medicaid fees to physicians and reimbursements to hospitals and long-term care institutions were limited, and differentials between what the nonpoor paid and what states paid on behalf of the poor under Medicaid grew ever larger. As a consequence resources available for the care of the poor, relative to those available for the nonpoor, declined. Yet at the same time, fueled with "guaranteed" Medicare dollars for the care of the aged (and, after 1973, the disabled), the hospital sector expanded and new technology was added, thus increasing pressure for additional expenditures.

The economic significance of the health sector ever more manifest, an expanding number of economists were attracted to the emerging field of medical economics. Given the attitudes and biases many economists and other Americans held about the virtues of competition in restraining price increases and the effectiveness of the free market in allocating resources appropriately, there appeared to be a simple (if not simplistic) explanation for the rising prices and expenditures: market structure and market failure.[9] The high and rising prices presumably reflected the health sector's lack of competition in the delivery of care as well as the unnecessary utilization of services that stemmed from insurance arrangements that insulated the patient from the financial implications of increased utilization. They were also associated with fee-for-service arrangements that placed the individual physician in an ambiguous (if not conflict-of-interest) situation. After all, the intervention that might be of little or no benefit to the patient's health was of certain benefit to the physician's pocketbook. The physician who provided the service and derived the income was also the decision maker determining the need for the service. Thus the possibility of conflict of interest.

"Consumer sovereignty," an important concept in microeconomics and in the theory of functioning markets, was hardly to be found in the world of medicine. Patients were not "sovereign"; they accepted and tended to follow their physician's recommendations. Furthermore, because of the breadth and depth of insurance coverage, many patients did not have to balance the costs of care against the potential benefits (even if only marginal) of one more visit, one more test, and one more procedure. Many economists decried insurance programs that provided "first-dollar" coverage and/or full coverage after a minimal deductible, preferring cost-sharing arrangements that would increase patient costs at the time of service and, presumably, change patient behavior (though, it was to be hoped, not affecting the utilization of preventive services). In contrast, other economists focused their attention on physician, rather than patient, behavior and emphasized the importance of changing the incentive structure that physicians faced. Though recognizing that it would be far more difficult to alter organizational arrangements than to reduce insurance coverage, they believed that the benefits of the former would far exceed those of the latter.

In the interim, that is, before markets could be reconstructed and competition enhanced, there were continuing efforts at regulation. These did not meet with much success, but they presumably provided evidence that the body politic was concerned about growth in expenditures. Nevertheless, ineffective regulatory activities (as, for example, was generally the case with Certificate of Need efforts to control capital investments in the health field) carried a cost. They caused a backlash among all providers of care as well as among those who sought care. In addition, they were burdensome and added to administrative expenditures.

As discussed earlier, models of organizational arrangements that altered physician incentives already existed. These encompassed structures under which physicians practiced within a predetermined budget or dollar constraint. These organizational structures, known as prepaid group practices (PGPs), had been part of the American health landscape for many years. Though PGPs had displayed their effectiveness and survival power, only a small fraction of Americans was familiar with the characteristics of prepaid group practice and an even smaller fraction was enrolled in the relatively few PGPs that existed in the early 1970s. Many employers saw little reason to bother offering employees an additional insurance option, particularly one that was unfamiliar and hard to explain. Many Americans viewed PGPs as organizations that would interfere with the traditional doctor-patient relationship and were loath to become subscribers. Others (incorrectly) believed that they would not have a personal physician if they joined a

PGP, and that they would somehow be entering a world of mass-produced medicine and overfilled waiting rooms. There was little reason to expect PGPs to expand without some outside stimulus and without federal assistance.

The Development of Health Maintenance Organizations

In 1971 the Nixon administration was concerned about rising health care costs and interested in offering an alternative to the Health Security Act, which had been proposed by Senator Edward Kennedy and Representative Martha Griffiths of Michigan, both Democrats. Building upon Medicare, this legislation would have provided universal health insurance through a social insurance mechanism and would have controlled expenditures through adoption of a federal health budget. President Nixon endorsed an initiative modeled after the PGP and intended to assist the growth of organizations that would link insurance with the delivery of care. The President called for the development of health maintenance organizations (HMOs), a name designed both to emphasize a commitment to early diagnosis and prevention and to mute criticism from organized medicine, which was antagonistic toward prepaid group practice.[10] In the HMO (as in PGPs) a group of care providers would agree to deliver all covered health care services to individuals within a group of subscribers for a predetermined monthly premium. As both insurer and deliverer of care, the HMO would assume the risks entailed in guaranteeing care to the defined group of subscribers. The assumption of financial risk would encourage the HMO to seek out economies and efficiencies in the delivery of care and, thereby, reduce its costs. Once the premium had been paid, the financial threat to the individual or family budget was minimized, if not eliminated, since (in their early history) HMOs typically limited subscriber out-of-pocket expenses to modest co-payments (such as a small set fee for a physician visit), seldom had deductible or co-insurance charges, and thus did not rely on cost-sharing to reduce utilization.[11]

Kennedy-like universal and comprehensive national health insurance would have to wait, but the system reform component that

its advocates had long supported (the expansion of PGPs) was embraced, and the generic term "health maintenance organization" was
adopted.[12] In opting for this approach the administration was heavily
influenced by a Minnesota physician, Dr. Paul Ellwood, who at the
time was executive director of the American Rehabilitation Foundation and of the Sister Kenny Institute of Minneapolis. He provided a
theoretical rationale that helped convince the administration to depart
from fee-for-service and adopt a fixed payment approach such as capitation. His arguments that this would help contain health care expenditures by unleashing market forces and stimulating competition
between HMOs and thus providing incentives to control utilization
(especially of hospital care) came at an opportune time. In part, his
success may have been due to the high proportion of administration
appointees in the Department of Health, Education, and Welfare who
came from California and had encountered and in some cases belonged to the large and successful Kaiser Permanente health program.
Its reputation as a deliverer of high-quality health care at reasonable
premium costs was such that its subscriber base cut across racial, ethnic, and income lines.[13] While many easterners associated the PGP
waiting room with hospital outpatient "clinic" medicine, westerners
viewed the PGP (most notably, Kaiser) as a high-quality institution.

In the context of the new priority given to cost containment, Ellwood's theory and the direct experience of many Nixon officials made
it possible to advocate the enactment of HMO legislation that would
have been considered too radical by earlier administrations. It was possible to argue that since the HMO plan contracted for services with a
group of physicians or employed physicians on a salary basis (perhaps with a bonus arrangement related to the plan's economic performance), physicians' incomes would not be boosted by increases in utilization. Thus there would no longer be an economic incentive to
perform more procedures or to generate extra visits or additional days
of hospitalization. Instead, there would be an economic incentive to
reduce future utilization by providing preventive and early diagnostic
procedures. The resulting economic gains might be shared by personnel in the form of higher incomes or shorter hours, and moreover by
those who paid for and those who used services (employers and em-

ployees) in the form of lower premiums and/or a wider range of benefits. As we shall see, in for-profit HMOs, whose rapid growth reflected their access to capital, the economic gains were shared with stockholders.[14]

The HMO (as well as the prepaid group practice plan after which it was modeled) provided something conspicuously lacking in other parts of the health care system: an organization that guaranteed and arranged care, made certain the necessary care providers were available, and had an incentive to emphasize preventive services. No longer did the patient encounter individual physicians, each with his or her own specialty, each self-employed and operating under fee-for-service arrangements. Instead of that fragmented approach, subscribers met providers who operated under an organizational umbrella. The vast majority of Americans who were not members of HMOs could complain *about*, but not *to*, the American health care delivery system. The "system," after all, was an abstract construct; it had no officers or bylaws. The Post Office would surely return any letters bearing the address "Complaint Department, American Health Care System" to the sender stamped "No Such Address." In contrast, HMO members had an organization to which they could voice their complaints. Thus the difference between independent practitioners, reimbursed on a fee-for-service basis for the care they provided to patients who walked through the office doors, and an organization with a fixed income, budget, and contractual obligations to a defined population of subscribers (what statisticians and epidemiologists called a "denominator") cannot be exaggerated. The words "accountability" and "responsibility" were given operational content.

The President signed the Health Maintenance Organization and Resources Development Act on December 29, 1973. It provided technical assistance as well as grants and loans designed to enhance the development of HMOs. Nevertheless, it took a number of years (and many amendments to the original legislation) before HMOs began to expand and spread across the country. In part the delay was due to the fact that the original legislation defined such a comprehensive set of health care benefits and set such high standards of performance that potential federally recognized HMOs felt that they would not be able to compete in the marketplace against traditional insurers with more restricted benefits and lower premiums. In part it was also due to physicians, patients, and employers who viewed these new constructs with some suspicion and were unwilling to change traditional insurance arrangements and providers. As a consequence it took a decade and more before HMOs and their organizational successors exerted a substantial impact on American medicine. Yet it can be argued that the action taken in December 1973 opened the door to a fundamental change in the structure and organization of the United States medical care delivery system.

The significance of that structural change cannot be overstressed, perhaps especially to those too young to fully appreciate how health insurance operated before the "HMO revolution." In the past insurance companies had collected premium dollars and paid bills or reimbursed subscribers; they did not involve themselves in the organization of the health care delivery system. Except for those individuals enrolled in PGPs, subscribers could seek care and take their insurance to any physician or hospital. With the spread of HMOs and its broader successor, "managed care," patients and prospective patients gave up the right to choose from among all physicians in practice and were limited to those physicians in the particular organization. Although economists could argue that the earlier freedom (when combined with the insulation from price as a variable affecting utilization decisions) led to greater health care expenditures, many subscribers valued the choices that those earlier arrangements provided (especially so if the employer was paying the major part of the premium).[15]

Nevertheless, as a consequence of economic pressures, the organization of health care changed. Employers found ways to exert such pressures to induce employees to enroll in HMOs. Thus, for example, an employer paid the premium (or contributed a percentage) for the lowest-cost HMO and required the employee who wanted to join a different and more expensive HMO or stay with a fee-for-service option (presuming the employer offered more than one option) to pay the difference in rates. Some employees with chronic conditions valued their long-standing relationships with physicians who may have practiced in more expensive programs. Not only did such employees have to pay more, but when healthier subscribers left these more expensive options, premiums for those who remained increased and, in a process akin to competition between community- and experience-rating, prompted even more employees to leave. American medical leaders had long praised "continuity of care," considering it one of the strengths of American medicine.[16] This continuity now gave way to these new economic pressures.

HMO arrangements represented an important change in the traditional relationship between insurance and delivery systems. In general, health insurance, including Medicare, was modeled after private insurance (so much so that Medicare initially did not cover preventive services) and accepted the patterns and incentives of the existing delivery system. In sharp contrast, the health maintenance organization was designed to alter and adjust delivery system incentives and provider behavior in an effort to control costs (most especially by reducing hospital utilization).

In attempting to change provider behavior and to stimulate cost-efficient care, HMOs did not accept the prevailing patterns of resource allocation generated by those who delivered care (especially physicians) as a given. Instead, delivery and insurance were linked with the expectation that since the organization operated within a budget and therefore had an incentive to develop and utilize a financial control mechanism, there would be changes in behavior, delivery system priorities, and resource allocations. Financial controls would affect the supply of personnel and (most directly, if, as in Kaiser's case, the PGP owned its own hospitals) hospital beds, the utilization of ambulatory and hospital services, and the patterns of care and costs. HMOs had an inherent economic logic. As a model of a controlled system that operated within a budget, their significance extended far beyond the fact that they offered comprehensive protection to millions of enrollees.

It should be clear that the argument for the economic logic of PGPs and HMOs does not imply that in the real world these organizations achieved all their goals. In many cases, for example, the incentive to stress preventive services could not overcome long-standing traditions that underemphasized such interventions. Furthermore, skeptics (and accountants) could argue that the costs of nonacute preventive services had to be borne today while the benefits would accrue in the future and might well accrue to another HMO with whom the subscriber would then have a relationship, an argument similar to one made explaining why individual employers might "underinvest" in non-firm-specific on-the-job training efforts. Furthermore, it was possible that just as the fee-for-service system could lead to overutilization and to doing more than was required, the HMO construct had an incentive (perhaps not fully offset by the "medical ethic") to deny care and do less than was necessary or desirable. This might express itself in subtle ways: long waiting times for appointments, expensive tests or therapy postponed a bit too long or rationed through other mechanisms, hospital discharges a bit too early, and redefinition of the term "medically necessary." One can easily imagine a situation in which a patient who is told "this procedure isn't necessary" would be skeptical when he heard that from an HMO physician ("he took my money and now doesn't provide the service") and yet enthusiastic if he heard it from a fee-for-service physician ("he could make more money, but has my best interests at heart").[17]

These various concerns were real. Medicine, after all, is an art as well as a science; physicians and nurses must exercise judgment, and the predominant "culture" can and does influence behavior. While fee-for-service medicine could be profligate in its resource use, HMOs (especially as an increasing proportion became for-profit and beholden to stockholders) ran the risk of being parsimonious. As with so much of medicine (and, one might add, of many other human activities) there is a need for balance, a characteristic most avidly to be sought, in part, because it is so difficult to attain.

Heads of medical institutions, including deans of medical schools, understood the nature of group practice and were aware of the HMO legislation. Indeed, the significance of prepaid group practice was apparent to the dean of the Harvard Medical School well before Paul Ellwood "came to Washington." As early as 1968 Dean Robert Ebert was instrumental in creating—at great financial risk to the medical school and over considerable opposition from alumni who were practicing in and near Boston and were concerned that he was developing a formidable "competitor"—the Harvard Community Health Plan, the first PGP in Massachusetts designed to deliver high-quality medical care and provide a locus for teaching outpatient medicine. Nevertheless, it is likely that few medical educators fully appreciated the impact that the HMO act would have on the growth of HMOs, on medical school curricula, and on the subsequent relationship between medical education and the world of practice both in and outside their affiliated hospitals. This is quite understandable: who, after all, would have believed that the HMO act would lead to a legislated revolution? Who of us can predict the nature and the impact of a revolution in its earliest stages?

Efforts to Increase Access

Even as the Nixon administration was supporting the 1973 HMO legislation, the pressures to expand health insurance—to view Medicare as a stepping stone toward universal health insurance—continued. The Kennedy-Griffiths Health Security Act could be considered as Medicare for all. Though favored by many of the two sponsors' fellow Democrats, it did not gain the support of the Democratic leaders of the two finance committees that would have to endorse the legislation: Russell Long, the chairman of the Senate Finance Committee, and Wilbur Mills, the powerful chairman of the House Ways and Means Committee.[18] While committees that dealt with health issues could hold hearings on national health insurance, funding for such a program required new taxes, and that in turn gave the finance committees jurisdiction over the legislation. Even so, there was a developing consensus that a mechanism of some kind to achieve national health insurance needed to be developed, enacted, and implemented, and, furthermore, that the nation was close to accomplishing these tasks.[19]

It therefore was not entirely unexpected that in 1974 the Nixon administration proposed a Comprehensive Health Insurance Program (CHIP) and supported this national health insurance proposal in a serious manner. The legislation was noteworthy in making an important departure from previous social insurance proposals that were financed through taxes and that included the entire population in a single program. Instead, it mandated employers to provide insurance to their employees (while providing subsidies and assistance designed to fill in the gaps that would inevitably arise because some employers and employees could not afford to bear the associated costs). This approach preserved the existing financing system, although, as many observers would argue, that meant preserving the numerous inefficiencies already in place under employer-employee private insurance. To many that represented a fiscal weakness; to others, it represented a political strength. In fact, of course, these were not mutually exclusive conditions.

If the HMO act was the basis for a revolution in the organization and financing of medicine, it can also be argued that CHIP led to a revolution—or at least a watershed—in the approach to national health insurance (NHI). Though the legislation failed of enactment, every President who subsequently proposed some form of NHI has built on the original mandated concept embodied in the CHIP proposal. Furthermore, the CHIP philosophy was adopted and adapted by Senator Kennedy (the leading Senate supporter of national health insurance and, till then, a proponent of a social insurance approach) and Congressman Mills. They retained the mandating idea but altered a number of the administration's specifications, expanded the benefits, preserved (but reduced) the levels of cost-sharing, and fashioned a proposal that had the potential to attract support from the broad middle of both parties. The debate seemed to have moved beyond a battle between competing "principles" and instead involved technical matters that could be negotiated.

The summer of 1974 was a busy time for the various congressional committees with jurisdiction on health matters.[20] Nevertheless, the search for a politically acceptable compromise proved fruitless. The relevant committees did not act on the President's CHIP proposal, on Kennedy-Mills, or other alternatives (such as the AFL-CIO-backed social insurance approach or an AMA tax credit measure). No group was strong enough to get a positive vote on its proposal, yet every group could find allies to defeat some other group's proposal.

Part of the explanation for inaction surely lies in the fact that those who felt they would be adversely affected (for example, small businesses that feared they would have to bear new costs for their previously uninsured and underinsured employees) spoke out against the legislation.[21] Furthermore, neither the American public nor its legislative representatives had had an opportunity to digest the proposals and become educated, organized, and involved (after all, Medicare, a much simpler and less fractious piece of legislation, took the better part of a decade to move from proposal to enactment).

Finally and importantly, there were a number of members of Congress and organizations who continued to believe in a social insurance program (like Medicare and Social Security), one that raised the necessary funds through taxes and that made benefits available to all. They saw the mandated approach as a fundamental error, a program that would be inefficient because it retained private insurance companies and would rely on the private sector to meet what they regarded as public sector responsibilities. To them, meeting public needs through private institutions implied a weaker role for public accountability than was appropriate. Thus groups supporting a social insurance approach as well as supporters of a mandated approach who wanted the measure to have less cost-sharing and otherwise be "liberalized" chose to wait for the results of the 1974 election, firmly believing that the newly elected Congress would act on national health insurance in a more "liberal" fashion.[22]

Indeed, a more liberal Congress was elected, but by then the Watergate political crisis had diverted attention and energy away from legislative initiatives. Both the Nixon proposal and the Kennedy-Mills bill lay dormant as the Congress and the nation were consumed by the historic drama and its aftermath. President Nixon's successor, President Ford, spoke about the importance of universal insurance and called for action. Yet Congress did not act. And though in the late 1970s President Carter developed a proposal, again Congress did nothing. It was almost a full twenty years, under President Clinton, before the nation once again witnessed—though, unlike Medicare, was not organized to participate in—a serious discussion about a specific piece of legislation designed to achieve universal health insurance. As we know, the Clinton effort also failed. It is not an exaggeration to suggest that at no time has the nation come as close to enacting a national health insurance program as it did in 1974. The explanation for this phenomenon does not lie in a decline in the need for such a program, but, among other factors, in the change in the nature and quality of political discourse. National health insurance remained on the political agenda, but did not command the sense of urgency that it did in the late 1960s and early 1970s. This can be explained, at least in part, by the way events once again conspired to make costs and cost control (rather than access) the dominant health policy theme.[23] National health insurance would have to wait. Nonetheless, some, citing British and Canadian experience, believed that not only was NHI not a fiscal threat, but that a national health program with budget controls was the only effective way to contain costs. They argued that although NHI would increase access to care, this would lead to only a short-term increase in health expenditures. This increase might be as little as, perhaps, 5 percent because many patients without insurance were already receiving services whose costs were borne in numerous complex and administratively costly ways (including being shifted to other payers). They argued that though total health expenditures would increase modestly at first, in a few years there would be a crossover point after which expenditures, while still increasing, would fall below what the costs of the existing inefficient non-NHI insurance and delivery system would have entailed. National health insurance and budget control, they suggested, was the nation's best, indeed only, hope for effective and equitable cost containment.

Nevertheless, even if the theory about reduced expenditures in the intermediate run was correct, the argument was not helpful in dealing with the present short-run, all too real budget implications of rising prices and expenditures as well as with long-standing skepticism about cost projections for new programs. The argument that a new and expansive program would reduce expenditures seemed implausible (unless one understood the inefficiencies embedded in the system). To say NHI "was a tough sell" is to understate the problem.

It was easy to see that legislative and executive branch staffs would be drawn to the opposite (and traditional) argument that held that whatever the virtues of NHI, the nation simply could not afford such a program, at least until health care expenditures were contained through regulation, legislated system change, a more competitive market, and consequent cost control. These various analysts, advisers, and decision makers envisioned a substantial increase in demand for health care as a result of NHI and a resulting increase in both prices and utilization. They argued that such had happened after Medicare and Medicaid were implemented. They were not convinced that the problem with those two programs was that they were embedded in a larger health care system that was inefficient and not price-conscious, and therefore that a national health program that covered the entire system would likely have a different outcome. In their view government regulators would not be able to contain the pressures to increase budgets, and increased expenditures would not be offset by increases in efficiency and savings in administrative costs.

Finally, they argued that even if all the regulators and their regulations were effective and all the hoped-for savings and efficiencies did occur, NHI would have a negative impact on the federal budget since the enactment of universal insurance had to mean that in large measure public dollars would substitute for the private dollars already in the system. Clearly this would be the case if the nation adapted a tax-based social insurance approach. It would also be true (though to a lesser extent) in an employer-mandated approach that utilized subsidies, tax credits, and other devices to enhance compliance and universality. The political implication of growth in federal expenditures (even if accompanied with a more than equivalent decline in private expenditures) was not appealing. Surely, it seemed safer to avoid the adoption of a new system and of new taxes and instead rely on somehow muddling through. Since most Americans did have some protection against the costs of medical care, reliance on the existing system carried minimal political risk.

The concern about rising costs and expenditures was a matter of top priority. After all, national health expenditures (NHE) constituted an increasingly larger proportion of the GDP, and there were no signs of a slowdown in their rate of growth. In 1960 NHE accounted for 5.1 percent of GDP; by 1965 (even before the implementation of Medicare and Medicaid) the share had risen to 5.7 percent. By 1970 the proportion had increased to 7.1 percent; by 1985 it had reached 10.3 percent.[24]

Nor was this growth accounted for solely by increases in that part of national health expenditures that went to administration, research, and construction (matters that at least in theory were amenable to control through the appropriation process). Expenditures for personal health care services (roughly 90 percent of national health expenditures) were also growing rapidly, both in absolute terms and as a share of GDP. In 1960 personal health care service costs totaled nearly $24 billion. By 1965 the total rose to $35 billion, and by 1985 to $376 billion (all in current dollars). Per-capita expenditures rose more than twelvefold, from $124 in 1960 to $1,523 in 1985. These increases affected all Americans and, not surprisingly, were accorded a higher priority than the issue of the uninsured and underinsured, which directly impacted a much smaller number (around 15 percent) of Americans. The uninsured were a minority. Furthermore, they were "others": the poor, black, Hispanic, the unemployed, low-wage earners, those too old to work and too young for Medicare. Conversely, rising health care expenditures were a political issue: they were visible and they affected the budgets of individuals and families, of firms that contributed to employee health insurance benefits, and of local, state, and federal governments that paid premiums for their employees and that funded public health and entitlement programs.

Congress was especially aware of and sensitive to the ever-increasing influence of medical care on the federal budget and those of other levels of government. In 1965 public financing of national health expenditures had totaled $10 billion (with a federal share of $5 billion). By 1970 public financing totaled $28 billion ($18 billion from federal funds), and in 1985 reached a total of $174 billion (with $123 billion coming from the federal government). Furthermore, in largest measure, health expenditures were not discretionary. Medicare expenditures had increased from $5 billion in 1967 to $72 billion in 1985, and Medicaid had increased from $3 billion ($1.4 billion federal) to $37.5 billion ($22.7 billion federal) over the same period. Taken together, expenditures for the two programs had risen from $7.7 billion to $109.8 billion. The pressures of health care expenditures on the federal budget—they were absorbing an increasingly large share, having grown from 3 percent of the federal budget in 1960 to 13 percent in 1985—were real and mounting.[25]

The level of frustration—what can we do, what do we do—was growing. The ongoing increase in health expenditures made it ever more difficult to fund other social initiatives. In ritualistic fashion legislators spoke about graft and corruption, and some suggested shifting costs to other levels of government and/or to beneficiaries and recipients. Yet, even as they offered these "quasi" answers, decision makers in government and in the private sector knew that they had no politically viable answer and that next year's health expenditures and share of GDP would exceed this year's. With an expanding and aging population and with advances in medical science and in the medical community's ability to intervene successfully (and not only in life-threatening situations), there was no reason to anticipate that expenditures would level off (either in absolute terms or as a percentage of federal and state budgets and employer expenditures for compensation).

Nevertheless, though cost issues continued to command attention, they could not entirely displace the problem of the uninsured. The uninsured, after all, were real people, not inanimate and somewhat abstract dollars. Furthermore, while Washington hearing rooms might ignore uninsured men and women and their children, that was not the case at the local level. There the various health care facilities had to provide services and had to be concerned about reimbursements and survival. They could not ignore the fact that America had an employment-based health insurance system, yet not all Americans were employed, nor did all employed Americans have access to insurance through their employer. They were painfully aware that the availability of insurance and, importantly, the level of employer contribution to premiums depended on factors such as the firm's geographic location, industry characteristics, number of employees, level of wages, and union strength.

In 1977, for example, over 99 percent of workers in firms with over 1,000 employees had access to an employment-related health insurance plan, compared with only 55 percent of workers in firms with twenty-five or fewer employees.[26] The problem, therefore, was not simply that employment-related group insurance tended to leave out individuals who were not employed, but that it was distributed unequally even among those who were. In general, workers in smaller and nonunionized firms (who usually had lower incomes) were less likely to have employment-related group coverage. Thus, even as the Carter administration felt that it had to focus on the control of health care costs (and especially hospital costs, which were the largest single element in the health care dollar), it was forced to address the problem of the distribution of insurance.

Given the system already in place and the large money flows involved, the Carter administration searched for a national health insurance structure that would retain the public-private mix that existed but extend its benefits more widely. It was felt that such an approach would minimize the disruption that a fully government-funded program would entail. It was also hoped that such a course would reduce political opposition. Not surprisingly, the administration turned to the mandated approach that had been developed in the Nixon administration.

Inevitably—and appropriately—the design of a universal health insurance program must be viewed as a political issue, one that cannot be approached merely as a technical problem in which "experts" search for the "best" technical solution to each administrative issue. Every prior decision to support or to reject a particular program (including the decision to exclude health insurance from the original Social Security program enacted in the Franklin Delano Roosevelt administration in 1935) had been a meld between the technical and the political.[27] So, too, it was (and had to be) in the Carter administration. The political advantages of retaining an important role for private insurance and an equally important one for employers appeared persuasive. Because Presidents and Presidential nominees who followed Carter also pursued a mandated approach (even while, as in President Clinton's case, stating that a social insurance approach was more efficient and less expensive), it is useful to elaborate on some of these matters.

Various Presidents have been influenced to retain the private insurance sector instead of shifting all money flows to the federal government because doing so would reduce the impact of health care and of health care inflation on the federal budget. Even if national health insurance expenditures would not increase the federal deficit because the program would be self-financed, there was no escaping the arithmetic: they would increase the share of federal expenditures within the GDP. President Carter had pledged to reduce that percentage, not expand it. Moving funds and expenditures from the private sector into government would hardly assist in meeting that commitment. Yet, if the dollars involved in NHI were not to flow through federal coffers, another body would have to serve as the conduit. The obvious candidates were the private insurers who, after all, were already receiving billions of dollars, who (in many cases) were administrative agents for Medicare, and who had the equipment and personnel to handle these and other administrative matters. Thus there was an additional justification (beyond their powerful political "special interest" status) for retaining private insurers and for assigning them a large role in any future program. Their retention seemed advantageous both in terms of politics and economics, a "win-win" situation.

In 1976 the Subcommittee on Health and the Environment of the House Committee on Interstate and Foreign Commerce issued *A Discursive Dictionary of Health Care.* The volume explained various terms used in the health care field. The entry for "National Health Insurance" read: "A term not yet defined in the United States."[28] In fact, of course, there were multiple definitions that kept changing as the goals that NHI was designed to achieve were modified, as new constraints arose, and as new programs were proposed. The Carter administration, like the Nixon administration a decade earlier and as the Clinton administration would do a decade later, rejected the definition of NHI as a single universal tax-based social insurance program. Instead, national health insurance was conceived of as a number of funding streams, each associated with and providing for different groups in the population. Minimizing the impact on the federal budget was so important that it justified the resulting administrative complexity that inevitably would add to health care system costs. Universality, it was hoped, would be assured by elimination of any uncovered population group; every American would be a member of a group that was included in one of the various programs. Presumably, the resulting patchwork quilt of America's health care coverage would work. All that was needed were a sufficient number of patches to cover everyone.

Under this approach most Americans would be covered by a private insurance sector that would expand in response to the requirement that employers provide protection for their employees. It was hoped that employers would not view the mandated premium as a disguised tax increase. Even so, there were important and direct implications for federal expenditures (and thus potentially for federal taxes): an increase in federal expenditures would be necessary in order to provide assistance to those who were not employed, worked in low-wage industries, or whose medical expenditures were likely to be above average. Furthermore, the lower the cost-sharing requirements and the broader the scope of benefits, the higher the premiums required. In turn, the higher the premiums, the more federal assistance would be required. Conversely, a program that reduced these impacts by setting minimal standards for insurance benefits could hardly be considered a significant accomplishment.

The search for a way to avoid having to choose between comprehensive (but costly) and inexpensive (but minimal) benefits led the Carter administration to advocate a "phasing" approach. Joseph Califano, the Secretary of the Department of Health, Education, and Welfare (HEW), testified that "with few exceptions, the consensus among legislators is that the 96th Congress cannot and will not digest a complete National Health Plan in one bite. The overwhelming number of those who favor eventual adoption of a National Health Plan urged me to bring this message back to the President: Ask the President to limit his legislative recommendation to the first phase of a National Health Plan and to describe his vision of a total plan so we can put that phase in context."[29] Secretary Califano's view that Congress would need two or more bites to digest a complete plan was at variance with an earlier statement ascribed to Sir Winston Churchill: "one doesn't leap over a chasm in two steps."

President Nixon had replaced "national" with "comprehensive" in his Comprehensive Health Insurance Plan; President Carter returned to "national," but dropped "insurance," and presented a National Health Plan that would be enacted and implemented in stages over an unspecified time. Importantly, there was no "trigger mechanism," no timetable for later action. Benefits and coverage would be limited at first but could be expanded in the future if Congress and whatever administration was in office at that time saw fit. There was no guarantee that would occur.

Senator Kennedy and organized labor, working through and with the Committee for National Health Insurance,[30] undertook the development of an alternative proposal. They searched for a design that would meet the President's requirements (minimal impact on the budget and a role for private insurance carriers). Furthermore, they faced their own requirement: that, though most of the funds in the system would flow in as private dollars, the system would enhance progressivity and redistribute dollars and services to low-income individuals and families. The construction of a progressive but partly private, partly public, program was a time-consuming and intricate undertaking.

The designs that emerged, one submitted by the administration and one sponsored by Senator Kennedy, the Health Care for All Americans Act (which rejected phasing), were very different but had two important similarities: both were exceedingly complex and worthy of Rube Goldberg,[31] and neither was as comprehensive (in a sense as "liberal") as the original Kennedy-Griffiths social insurance approach, President Nixon's initiative in 1974, or the Kennedy-Mills bill response to that initiative. Though both were Democrats, President Carter, the party leader, and Senator Kennedy, the leading proponent of national health insurance, were unable (or unwilling) to compromise their differences on NHI. When it became clear that those who favored NHI could not agree on a single bill that could command their support, the chances for favorable action disappeared. The history of NHI has often exhibited this characteristic: agreement on the importance of universal coverage, disagreement on how to reach that goal, and, as a consequence, inaction.

Health care costs and expenditures continued to increase. Employers and employees with health insurance faced higher premiums; costs of care for those who could not pay continued to be shifted to individuals with health insurance; Medicare beneficiaries could see a widening gap between physicians' actual fees and those approved by Medicare; state legislators faced the budgetary effects of rising Medicaid expenditures. In response, the Carter administration advocated more regulation (in particular, of hospital prices). This effort was rejected by members of Congress who wanted to reduce health care expenditures but feared that price regulation would reduce the quality of care and/or would impact unfavorably on their local community hospitals. Furthermore, government regulations were increasingly coming under attack as interference with the market. There were more and more calls for removal of restrictions that interfered with and inhibited market competition.

The argument that a national health insurance program with a tight budget would help contain costs may have impressed some academic analysts, but few legislators felt at ease with a budgeting system that Secretary Patricia Harris, whom President Carter had selected as Secretary Califano's successor, had testified "is beyond our technical capability . . . could work only in a highly structured health system which places severe limits on consumer access . . . [and] would inevitably result in an arbitrary rationing of health care services."[32] Furthermore, adoption of national health insurance would have injected government into matters that lay in the private sector and for which physicians, hospitals, and insurance carriers (but not members of Congress) were held responsible. Thus, faced with the intractable economics of the health care arena, the Carter administration gave priority and attention to dual and, in part, contradictory efforts to enhance both regulatory efforts and competitive initiatives that might help contain cost and expenditure increases. If one medicine would not work, why not add another?

Medicine Becomes a Growth "Industry": An Overview

The rapid increase in medical interventions as a result of scientific advances, the addition of personnel and facilities, the expansion of private health insurance, and the implementation of Medicare and Medicaid, led to significant increases in health expenditures (both in absolute dollars and as a percentage of the Gross Domestic Product). The combination of knowing more about what to do, having the resources to do it, and the lowering of financial barriers to having it done, added dollars to the medical care system. And the inevitable heightened efforts to deal with these price and expenditure increases led to new ways to organize the delivery of medical care, to managerial complexity that over time would create many new problems, and to the "regulatory revolution." In turn, some of the failures of the regulatory approach, failures that arose because of the inherent tension between regulation and the free market, led to subsequent efforts at deregulation. In responding to this tension medicine was subject to the same forces found in other arenas, for example, airlines and telecommunication.

Nevertheless, the attention devoted to these various problems does not negate that, on balance, changes in the decades following World War II (the period from 1945 to 1985), including the policies adopted at various levels of government, served the nation extraordinarily well. They resulted in a number of successes. At the end of World War II, for example, America faced a shortage of health care personnel, a deficiency of acute-care hospital beds, and a relatively inadequate level of total health expenditures. All of these problems were corrected (indeed, overcorrected).[33] Importantly, the nation's medical and public health efforts not only increased resource inputs, and availability and access to care, but also improved health outcomes. Various indicators such as life expectancy, infant mortality rates, and morbidity and mortality rates from acute infectious diseases improved significantly. The sharp reduction in mortality from heart disease and stroke was especially striking.

As the decade of the 1980s was beginning it seemed clear that we were on the threshold of emerging new problems bred by these very successes. Policy makers, health care professionals, hospital administrators, and the public had little experience with an adequacy of resources. Regrettably, the medical community and public officials (responding to lobbying efforts by "experts" in white coats and wanting to help medicine while unwilling to address universal health insurance) behaved as though we still had deficits. The United States was growing, and incomes and the standard of living were improving. It was easy and natural to assume further growth and to plan within an ethos of expansion that had come to be considered as synonymous with progress. "More" was assumed to be "better," and few considered the balance between health expenditures and other social needs, whether we were getting value for money, or whether the additional dollars were going to the areas of highest medical need.

There was little awareness of or willingness to address the need to equilibrate the system, to provide appropriate services for all Americans (including the poor and the uninsured), and to redress the imbalance between the distribution of services: specialist and generalist, urban and rural, poor and affluent. Instead of fine-tuning the system and redistributing resources, we continued to expand total inputs. It was as if we believed that if we flooded the system with more practitioners, more technology, more resources of all kinds, and, above all, more dollars, some of the resources would necessarily flow to the areas of need (and that, somehow, the nation could absorb the accompanying waste and not be troubled by it). It was as if the "trickle down" theory found application in medicine, and with the same lack of efficacy as in other areas of civic life!

The rapid increase in the flow of dollars came to be expected and created an altered attitude toward further growth. Hospitals and other health care institutions, oblivious to the questions "What does the community need?" and "How much is enough?" and desiring to upgrade their own facilities, assumed debt obligations to finance expansion, debt obligations that they believed would be repaid out of "guaranteed" Medicare, supplemented by Medicaid and private insurance dollars. Rashi Fein recalls how a hospital general director described the change that resulted from the new flow of government funds. He stated that in pre-Medicare/Medicaid days he had a list of new devices that the medical staff wanted, and so he tried to match items on that list with prospective donors. With the advent of Medicare/Medicaid, the list disappeared: a wealthy donor, a member of the family, one Uncle Sam, had appeared. The hospital director no longer found it as necessary to solicit philanthropists. Guided by self-interest rather than community needs, every institution projected increases in market share and based its decisions on these—mutually inconsistent—projections. Presumably, the laws of arithmetic had been repealed. In the private sector, institutions that once had been community enterprises, supported by charitable giving, now became mega-centers whose expansion was made possible by the sale of bonds. But the principal and interest had to be repaid. Consequently, medical care had to count on a continuing increase in dollars. The objective became one of keeping the beds filled and the flow of research grants sustained.[34]

Inevitably, there was less pressure to discharge the patient who for personal reasons wanted to stay an extra day in the hospital (perhaps it would be more convenient for a family member to bring the patient home a day later), or whose physician wanted to feel a bit more comfortable and exhibit his or her concern by keeping the patient in hospital a bit longer. Yielding to these pressures not only meant additional revenue to the institution, but since these "healthier" patients needed less care, they were more profitable. The hospital could claim it had increased efficiency, since the average cost of care declined even as the total costs and expenditures increased. Such criteria ignored the societal impact and suggested that the most efficient and profitable hospitals would be those that rejected the sickest patients and admitted only healthier ones. Such behavior would run contrary to the purposes of the medical care system. Nevertheless, we shall find that as a consequence of the "entrepreneurial revolution" that followed the period under discussion, hospitals (especially those owned by for-profit entities) did shun the sickest patients, and insurance companies did try to enroll healthier subscribers. "Cream skimming" and "cherry picking" became more common. The quest for profits was an imperative.

It was becoming clear to the federal government (which was paying for all of Medicare and a very substantial part of Medicaid) and to private insurers and third-party payers that hospital payment (akin to physician fee-for-service payment) operated under a set of perverse incentives. Payers needed to develop payment policies (commonly called "reimbursement") that would help constrain system expenditures. As a result in fiscal 1984 Medicare began to phase in a new reimbursement system under which hospital payment would no longer be the product of "reasonable" per diem costs multiplied by the number of patient days of care (plus extras for nonordinary costs, such as operating rooms or x-rays). Instead, the Health Care Financing Administration defined 467 diagnostic categories and reimbursed hospitals a predetermined number of dollars per patient having a particular diagnosis. As time went on, this Diagnosis Related Group (DRG) system was fine-tuned and became more detailed and more responsive to important institutional characteristics. Since various adjustment factors (such as geographic location, area wage rate, and cost of medical education) were taken into account, hospitals did not each receive the same amount per diagnosis. Nevertheless, each institution had an incentive to search for efficiency and to conserve resources, since the fixed amount it would receive per diagnosis was known in advance.

The incentives that a set price provides as a stimulus to efficiency were obvious. So, too, however, were the dangers posed to the quality and distribution of care. In a situation analogous to fee-for-service as contrasted with capitation, the traditional hospital per diem payment might provide incentives to overtreatment, but the fixed price might lead to undertreatment and rapid discharge. Some hospitals, in fact, encouraged physicians to inform patients that they had "used up" the number of days on which the particular DRG was based. Though this was operationally meaningless since no Medicare beneficiary faced an arbitrary hospital limit on necessary services, many patients feared that they would be discharged. Additionally, when there were multiple medical problems (as was often the case for both aged and/or disabled Medicare patients) hospitals had an incentive to define as the primary diagnosis the condition whose "fixed price" would prove most profitable. Indeed, some hospital corporations were charged in the courts for having done this, and have made multimillion-dollar settlements with the government as a consequence.[35] Furthermore, though the system of payment attempted to deal with "outliers," that is, patients who needed considerably more care than the average on which the fixed rate was based, the DRG payment might not take full account of severity of illness. Thus there was an incentive to shun patients who were very ill and whose costs of care were likely to exceed the level of payment.

The risks in any payment system are apparent. The way dollars flow changes incentives and therefore behavior. The protection that the individual and the community had against too much economizing lay in consumer awareness, the traditional medical ethos, and the efficacy of vigorous government review and oversight, activities that require a belief in government and governmental regulation as well as sufficient funding to accomplish the supervisory mission. In the early 1980s the question was whether the public would be able to count on an executive and legislative commitment to provide funding required to conduct the necessary regulatory and review activities. Moreover, was the consumer sufficiently knowledgeable and willing to speak up, and could the medical ethos remain sufficiently strong in the face of the growth of for-profit institutions that were beholden to stockholders, the ever-increasing emphasis on market economics, and the entrepreneurial revolution that was underway. Not unexpectedly, stockholders and bondholders looked for dividends and interest, not for the psychic rewards of doing good. Furthermore, the traditional view that the patient would be protected by the physician serving as the patient's advocate was being eroded as physicians came under increasing economic pressures applied by those for whom they worked or by insurance companies and their payment criteria.

Hospitals, of course, have varying missions. They are sponsored and supported in different ways (government, community-at-large, medical school and university, religious denominations). Some are profit-oriented and investor-owned. Most are not-for-profit institutions. Where they still exist, public city and county hospitals continue to serve all patients, including those "dumped" by other institutions. In many hospitals the trustees' sense of a community service mission and the staff's ethical standards protect and can be expected to continue to protect against undesirable side-effects. Nevertheless, there has been reason for concern. As hospital budgets grew tighter, as the search for efficiency evolved into a consuming priority, and as an increasing proportion of hospitals answered to stockholders or bondholders rather than to the general community, power necessarily shifted to financial administrators. When the hospital became a "business" and clinical divisions became "profit centers," there was an inevitable temptation and pressure to cut back on free care and community obligations. The justification—and it was not a trivial justification, given the American health care system and its organization and funding characteristics—

was the need for a favorable bottom line. The need to survive and the desire to flourish were vital and sometimes called for a reassessment of the hospital's sense of mission.

These were not matters or issues that affected only the for-profit institutions. In a world of competition, in a world in which third-party payers wanted to reduce payment levels and in which employers wanted to minimize their insurance costs, not-for-profit institutions were forced to similar standards of behavior as their competitors. They could not ignore the bottom line; they could not rely solely on good will; they were forced to behave as if they were seeking a profit. In that world the desire to maximize the amount that revenues exceed expenditures (which even not-for-profits called "profit") trumped all other cards.

As noted, as health expenditures escalated and further growth was anticipated, opportunities to reap financial rewards were apparent, and a for-profit delivery system emerged and grew rapidly. The dollars were there: financed with Medicare, Medicaid, and private health insurance. Though all would proclaim the need for and the importance of cost control, there was reason to believe that health care expenditures would continue to escalate and that for-profit health institutions could deliver a high rate of return on investment dollars. Constraints on total expenditures were relatively few and weak, and many institutions (including newly emerging ones) wanted their "share of the pie." Health care services corporations moved onto Wall Street as financiers came to recognize financial opportunities. Those who received dollars wanted more, and those who financed care still believed in the deficit model or felt that there was no way to slow the flow of dollars without running the risk of reducing the quality and availability of care and, therefore, reversing the improvement of the nation's health or at the minimum risking public opprobrium if untoward events could be attributed to "penny pinching." Those in charge of allocating dollars and setting reimbursement rates hesitated to provoke the political hazard of disappointing a public that seemed to believe that more dollars translated into health improvement.

Nor was it clear how expenditures could be controlled. Regulation had not been particularly efficacious, and the argument that it had been too tepid (rather than too strong) was at variance with the deregulation movement that began during the Carter administration. The "climate of opinion" appeared to call for reliance on market forces, but no one knew how to turn the spigot down and reduce the flow of government and private sector dollars that were underwriting growth and expansion.

The response to the deficit model that had dominated health policy during the two decades of the post–World War II period had been a striking increase in expenditures for health care services. By the mid-1970s voices were raised about impending surpluses of health care resources, especially in relation to acute-care general hospital beds and health care professionals. Simplistic notions about how to contain costs were floated. In a reversal from reliance on government price-setting and regulation, "competition" was embraced by many as the panacea, and reliance on the free market, which would "unleash" competitive forces, and lead to growth in productivity and to moderation in price increases, became "the" answer. Obsessed with price competition, the Federal Trade Commission believed that competition would be stimulated and price increases moderated if physicians were permitted to advertise. Until then, physicians held that advertising was unethical: discreetly modest announcements that Dr. So and So had moved to the community and was opening a practice pushed the limits beyond which physicians dared not go. Similarly, physicians (unlike dentists) felt that they could be accused of unethical solicitation of business if they sent out reminders that it was time for a checkup.

Rashi Fein remembers that in a quest for subscribers during the early days of the Harvard Community Health Plan, administrators wanted to advertise the existence of this new prepaid group practice, but plan physicians objected that this might lead to charges of unethical behavior on their part. That was an earlier time; now traditional modes of behavior, attitudes, and standards were changing. The health professions proved no match for the financial forces that came to dominate health policy. Articles began to appear on the "corporatization and the social transformation of doctoring,"[36] on the "monetarization of medical care,"[37] and "is medicine a business or a profession?"[38]

Old, well-understood, and stable relationships could no longer be relied on. The infrastructure of medicine, its financial and organizational patterns, was being modified. Physicians and other health professionals had to deal with and accommodate new forces and new pressures. And likewise the health institutions that trained the health care labor forces (most especially, the schools of medicine and of public health) also had to adapt to these new conditions.

4 | Education for the Health Professions: The Impact of Growth

Health care and the nation's health status are dependent on many factors. Important as health insurance and access to health care services are, they are only two of many variables affecting the health of the population, and thus only two of the many variables with which all administrations should be concerned. It is easy to focus on the various economic arrangements in health care because they are important, the subject of government activity, and the center of media attention. That focus, however, makes it easy to overlook the purpose of the various economic arrangements and of the economic activity in health care. That purpose is the improvement of the health of individuals and of the population.

Economic arrangements do influence the behavior of key participants in the health enterprise arena. It is also true, however—and needs to be stressed—that this enterprise is indeed about health, and that health and health care are "different" and are viewed differently than other goods and services. These differences, in turn, influence the possible economic arrangements. As we do not subscribe to the view that "you don't have to know the subject matter as long as you know how to teach," so we do not subscribe to the view that "you do not have to know that the subject is health care as long as you know how markets work." Therefore, we need to ask what changes were taking place to health and health care while Washington was preoccupied with health expenditures and, to a lesser extent, with access.

Improvements in the Public's Health

During the Carter administration Julius Richmond had the opportunity to serve simultaneously as the Assistant Secretary for Health in the Department of Health, Education, and Welfare (renamed the Department of Health and Human Services in 1979) and as Surgeon-General of the United States Public Health Service (USPHS). Several trends in the improvement of the public's health could be identified,

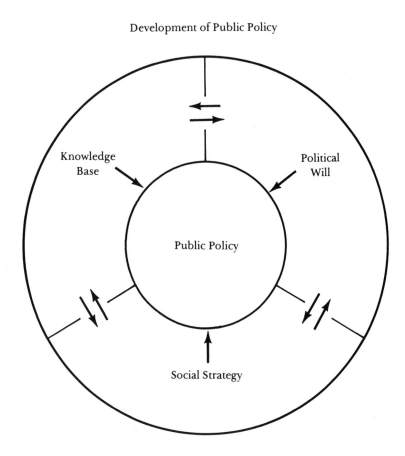

Development of Public Policy

Figure 2. Three-Factor Approach to Health Policy. *Source:* From J. B. Richmond and M. Kotelchuck, "Political Influences: Rethinking National Health Policy," in C. H. McGuire et al., *The Handbook of Health Professions Education* (San Francisco: Jossey-Bass, 1983).

and it was clear that to further these improvements three ingredients were required: a rich and expanding knowledge base, a social strategy for the application of that knowledge base, and the political will to implement that social strategy and thus apply the knowledge base. This is expressed in Figure 2, which provides the conceptual analytic model for examining the interacting forces shaping public policy.

A number of these improving trends, already apparent in the mid-1980s and continuing to the present, can be summarized. There has been a significant increase in longevity over the last century.[1] United States life expectancy at birth has gone from 49.2 years in 1900 to 76.9 years in 2000. Although many demographers had previously believed that it was unlikely that life expectancy at age sixty-five years and older would improve, it has become evident that the most rapidly growing segment of the population is, in fact, the eighty-five years and older population group.[2] Consequently, while the total United States population tripled during the period 1900 to 2000, the number of individuals sixty-five and over grew by a factor of 11 and the number of those eighty-five and over grew by a factor of 33.

Contributing to the United States longevity data was the surprisingly large decline in mortality from heart disease and stroke. The former was cut from 587 per 100,000 persons in 1950 to 258 in 2000. The implications are quite dramatic: had the 1950 rates applied in the year 2000, there would have been a total of 1,651,000 deaths from heart disease. In actuality there were 725,000. A full 926,000 deaths had been averted. The death rate from stroke exhibited an even more dramatic rate of decline: from 180.7 per 100,000 in 1950 to 60.9 five decades later.[3] Many physicians had despaired about reducing mortality from diseases that are due to multiple causes. Yet the science base, the social strategy, and the appropriate political will resulted in policies that encouraged the public to begin to act on the growth in knowledge about the effects of diet, physical activity, smoking, stress, and early hypertension detection and treatment.

Though the rate of decline has been different, the United States infant mortality rate has also gone down over the last half century (and by 90 percent over the full century). This, too, was primarily the result of advances in public health along with improvements in clinical care.

Death rates for heart disease and stroke (and numerous other conditions) exhibit significant disparities by income, race, ethnicity, and rural-urban residence (matters that, as we shall indicate, increasingly are the subject of important epidemiological research). This is also true, embarrassingly so, of infant mortality, which has long exhibited persistent differentials and disparities. While the rate was 6.8 per 1,000 live births in 2001, the rate for whites was 5.7 and for blacks 10.2.[4] Furthermore, the United States rates are higher than those found in other industrialized countries and cannot be entirely explained by the higher rates found for blacks and Native Americans.

Even more embarrassment can arise in a comparison with other countries. It is apparent that we do not receive "value for money." Many countries spend as little as half of the percentage of their (often, lower) GDP on medical care as does the United States. Nevertheless, as Figure 3 demonstrates, it is possible for them to have lower infant mortality rates than we. The relationship between expenditures and infant mortality, even within the industrialized countries of the Organization for Economic Co-operation and Development (OECD), clearly shows that the United States is an outlier, underscoring the point made earlier that the nation's health status is dependent on many factors.

Many Americans (including many physicians) would have overlooked international comparisons and, focusing on the declines in United States death rates over time, would have ascribed these advances to the "miracles of modern medicine"—to our gleaming hospitals, increasing use of technology, expanding research budgets, and pharmaceutical investments. Nevertheless, a growing professional consensus held that the various health gains were largely the consequence of progress in applying our knowledge of health promotion and disease prevention rather than of improved clinical care. In a sense this was very similar to a much earlier time when advances in health could more properly be ascribed to improvements in living conditions (including, notably, sanitation) than to medical advances. While the importance of clinical care as a basic human need should not be minimized, it was apparent that the revolution in biology subsequent to World War II, a revolution that had brought many advances

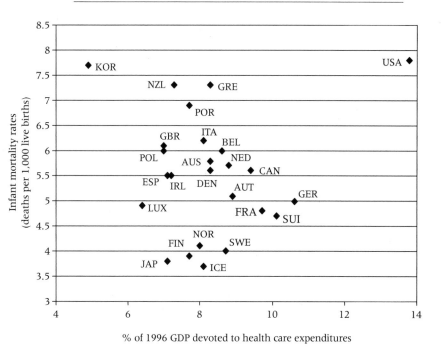

% of 1996 GDP devoted to health care expenditures

AUS = Australia	GRE = Greece	NZL = New Zealand
AUT = Austria	ICE = Iceland	NOR = Norway
BEL = Belgium	IRL = Ireland	POL = Poland
CAN = Canada	ITA = Italy	POR = Portugal
DEN = Denmark	JPN = Japan	ESP = Spain
FIN = Finland	KOR = S. Korea	SWE = Sweden
FRA = France	LUX = Luxembourg	SUI = Switzerland
GBR = United Kingdom	NED = Netherlands	USA = United States
GER = Germany		

Figure 3. International Comparison of Health Care as a Percentage of GDP and Infant Mortality Rates, 1996. *Source: OECD Health Data 2000: A Comparative Analysis of 29 Countries,* CD-ROM (OECD, 2000).

to clinical care, as yet had only marginal effects on our improving vital statistics.[5]

These trends and their origins became ever more evident during a period when increasingly powerful mathematical and statistical techniques were being developed. In this regard one cannot overemphasize the importance of the introduction of the desktop computer, which permitted and encouraged new subjects for, and modes of, analysis. A growing proportion of medical and public health students and investigators were applying the tools of epidemiology and bio-statistics. Evidence-based medicine (the awareness of the strength of the evidence supporting particular clinical practices) and the measurement of effectiveness and efficacy—in no small measure inevitable responses to rising costs and the need to justify medical interventions and investments in new capital equipment—were taking hold. Our improving understanding of these various trends and of their origins helped create a sense of optimism about the power of our expanding knowledge base in health promotion and disease prevention.

As a consequence of the application of more powerful statistical methodologies and the implications of this newfound knowledge, Dr. Richmond, as Surgeon-General, decided to develop and direct attention to a specific set of health goals for the nation and to the need to further expand the knowledge base, develop a social strategy, and mount the political will to attain those objectives. This process was advanced in 1979 by institutionalizing the creation of ten-year targets through the development and release of a report, *Healthy People: The Surgeon-General's Report on Health Promotion and Disease Prevention*.[6] The quantitative goals that were incorporated had been developed by a consensus conference, held under the auspices of the staff of the Centers for Disease Control and Prevention, and were published as a companion volume under the title *Promoting Health, Preventing Disease: Objectives for the Nation*.[7]

Significantly, this was designed not to be a one-time effort; the process has been repeated at ten-year intervals by subsequent Surgeons-General. The resulting decennial reports have become road maps for improving public health.[8] Their importance has been immeasurably increased because they are not mounted as an "in-house" product.

Rather, they involve multiple citizen constituencies as well as extramural health professionals whose contribution in setting goals and in aiding in and assessing and monitoring progress toward their achievement is significant. Furthermore, as contributors to this activity, they have an interest, a vested stake, in disseminating findings and in supporting efforts designed to help attain the various objectives.

The Growth of Schools of Public Health

The mounting public interest in health promotion was reflected in the founding and expansion of schools of public health, whose research, demonstration, and teaching programs were focused on the health of populations. Their missions contrasted sharply with those of medical schools, which emphasized individual clinical care. Early in the twentieth century there had been a growing recognition of the importance of public health and a growing dissatisfaction with the perceived inadequacy of the medical schools in providing education for that field. With support from the Rockefeller Foundation, the Johns Hopkins School of Hygiene and Public Health was founded in 1913. By 1958 there were eleven accredited schools of public health, with a total enrollment of under 1,200 students. By 2003 there were thirty-three schools with over 19,000 students. These schools are much larger (mean enrollment has grown from slightly over 100 students per school in 1958 to over 575 in 2003). Their student bodies are also much more diverse: two-thirds of the students are female, one-third is of minority group background, and one-sixth is foreign.[9]

With the expanding understanding and application of epidemiology and statistics, faculty members in schools of public health (including an increasing number of social scientists) became more involved and prominent in the shaping of health policy and in issues involving finance, organization, and the administration of health sector institutions.[10] These newer interests were joined to long-standing traditional interests in such matters as clean water, sewage disposal, and other aspects of the environmental infrastructure that directly and visibly affect the public's heath. This development presented new opportunities for social scientists who wanted to specialize in applying their disciplines to the study of health affairs. The faculties of schools of public health represented a broader range of interests and frequently had stronger ties to their counterparts in the faculties of arts and sciences than to colleagues in the schools of medicine. Their agendas took explicit account of the fact that "population health," the enhancement of the health of the population, required much more than a concern with the physical environment or with the summation of the results of clinical interventions on individual patients at the bedside or in the physician's office.

This statement of the different perspectives of medicine and public health should be taken as nonjudgmental. Clearly, both perspectives are valid. Just as it was important to add to our understanding of factors that influenced the health status of communities and their members and to undertake programs to improve health indicators, so too it was important to treat the individual patient in distress. It was as if the economist in public health knew about the "uninsured," but had never encountered an uninsured individual, while the practicing physician knew his uninsured patient, Mrs. Jones, but did not understand the more general phenomenon. Dealing with the real patient and dealing with the statistical general public required different (albeit, on occasion, overlapping) skills, and each was more than a full-time job. That was especially true as the scientific knowledge base exploded. Clinicians were understandably increasingly preoccupied with incorporating the many advances in clinical care rather than focusing on health promotion. The former had an immediate urgency, for the patient needed help; the latter could be postponed—the patient would still be there tomorrow.

In addition to the demands placed upon medical practitioners by the need to stay abreast of the many rapid advances in treatment (including new drugs and changing drug regimens), the increases in expenditures for medical care and growing regulations, paper work, and the inherent complexity of such tasks placed great emphasis on efficiency and on improving productivity. This combination of trends and stresses inevitably added to the time pressures under which practicing physicians worked and created frustration. It was difficult for clinicians to fulfill the various expectations they encountered: those of patients, chiefs of service, hospitals, colleagues, insurers, even their own families. On the one hand, medicine was ever more exciting as new procedures, technology, and knowledge expanded. On the other hand, clinicians were accused of ordering too many tests, doing too many procedures, and spending too much money. Although medical educators emphasized the importance of taking a complete history, understanding the social context, and listening to the patient, all of these required time, and time was the scarcest resource. Insurers tended not to reimburse for time but for procedures.

These various factors made it ever more difficult for practicing physicians to broaden their horizons. Thus the terrain was left to others, and the visibility and importance of the public health agenda were enhanced. Advances in our understanding of public health issues and the sharing of that knowledge through public health education occurred largely as a consequence of forces that lay, and actions taken, outside the traditional medical care system that incorporated the practitioner, his or her office, and the hospital. The United States Public Health Service (particularly through the Surgeon-General's *Report on Health Promotion and Disease Prevention*), state and local public health agencies, the large voluntary health organizations (such as the American Heart Association, the American Cancer Society, and dozens of others), the schools of public health, and (increasingly) the media devoted more and more attention to public health education. These efforts helped create a climate for changes in health behaviors. As a consequence even the politically powerful tobacco industry, with enormous resources to counter the various health messages, witnessed a steady decline in cigarette smoking.

That decline is an excellent example of how research contributed to an improved knowledge base concerning the various health hazards associated with cigarettes and with the effects of passive smoking, how that knowledge base and additional research contributed to the development of a social strategy to reduce the habit, and how the political will required to alter behavior (and materially affect the social acceptability of smoking) was created and strengthened.

In the early decades of the century the increase in cigarette smoking, especially among males, resulted in the greatest man-made epidemic in history, that of lung cancer. By midcentury, in 1964, research demonstrating the link between smoking and lung cancer was sufficiently compelling to enable the Surgeon-General, Dr. Luther Terry, to issue a definitive report of his Advisory Committee on Smoking and Health.[11] There was documentation of the effects of smoking on other conditions, such as heart and cardiovascular disease. Subsequently, additional research documented the dangers of passive smoking, thus adding concern about the impact of smoking on the public at large to the earlier concern about the consequences to the individual smoker. In spite of very considerable expenditures by the tobacco industry in efforts to deny the relationships between smoking and health,[12] the combined educational efforts of public health agencies and voluntary health organizations have resulted in a gradual decline in the annual per capita consumption of cigarettes, from 4,345 cigarettes per capita among Americans eighteen years and older in 1963 to 2,082 cigarettes per capita in 2000.[13]

The Growth of Medical Centers

Physicians and patients who have grown up in what some consider the golden age of medicine would most probably be shocked to discover that prior to World War II physicians had little by way of specific therapies for their patients. The general public and even today's younger health professionals would surely be astonished to learn that a review of medical textbooks of the 1930s, when one of us was a medical student, indicates that the only specific medical therapies then available were liver extract for pernicious anemia, insulin for diabetes, quinine for malaria, arsenicals and heavy metals for syphilis, and digitalis for heart failure. Today's sophisticated imaging and diagnostic techniques, pharmaceutical interventions, transplantation, and microsurgery techniques did not exist. The medical and surgical resources were extremely limited.

The availability of antimicrobial medications, initially that of sulfonamides, just prior to World War II, transformed the treatment of the infectious diseases. It also created a hopeful climate for intensifying and expanding medical research during and after the war. The time was ripe, therefore, for the rapid growth of the National Institutes of Health (NIH) and the creation of a remarkably inventive partnership between the federally funded NIH and the private and state universities and research institutions of the nation.[14] As a consequence of the increased complexity of medical care and expansion in the flow of research funds, academic medical centers that could deal with that complexity and that were equipped to respond to the research opportunities and to the availability of funds with which to undertake them, underwent rapid expansion.

In the process, research came to play a much more important role for individual medical school faculty members—both in relation to their allocation of time and to the criteria applied for promotion. The academic medical centers came to be increasingly characterized as a three-legged stool made up of research as well as teaching and patient care. While medical educators were intensely concerned that federal dollars to provide general support to their schools and educational missions might lead to political intrusion into issues in education, similar concerns were not generally present (certainly not as intensely) in the case of federal funding for research. Instead, there was a feeling of strong partnership between the medical schools, their affiliated teaching hospitals, and the National Institutes of Health.

The Institutes provided healthy support for basic sciences in general as well as for the specific areas of Institute responsibility. Lobbying by advocacy groups for appropriations on behalf of particular programs (what might be called "special interest" lobbying that was at variance with the academic scientists' desires to set scientific priorities) had the effect of lifting all boats. The pluralism of the lobbying efforts turned out to be quite compatible with the interests of the scientific community. NIH appropriations grew substantially and remarkably: from $773 million in 1966, to over $2 billion in 1975, and to over $5 billion by 1985.[15]

In largest measure, faculty members from across the country determined the expenditure of appropriated federal funds through a system of governance involving scientific committees ("study sections"), councils (including public representatives) of the various Institutes, and (more recently) the Director's Council of Public Representatives (which includes, among others, representatives of voluntary health associations). The flow of federal funds to the universities caused many faculty members to have greater feelings of loyalty to the granting agencies than to their universities—a matter that led university administrators to have a measure of ambivalence about the flow of federal dollars.[16]

The leadership of medical centers often was slow to recognize the need for organizational change to accommodate the rapid institutional growth and associated increased complexity. This was described by David Rogers, the former dean of the Johns Hopkins School of Medicine and later president of the Robert Wood Johnson Foundation, who wrote about the dysfunction of older organizational arrangements. He presented a chart with the design of an effective and responsive organization: an individual at the top, four persons reporting to him, and four persons reporting to each of those four. In contrast he drew a picture of the design of a medical school: one person at the top, and some twenty-two persons at an equal level reporting to the one dean.[17]

The commitment of the university medical centers to clinical care and clinical investigation provided an essential component of, and stimulus to, the rapidly expanding science base. In turn, this commitment contributed to improved patient care. The emerging developments in genetics, molecular biology, immunology, and imaging methods made the teaching hospitals and their outpatient departments essential for the care of patients with complex, serious illness. The individual consultant found that he or she could no longer function in isolation. In the best of worlds, and a number of medical centers embodied the best of worlds, house staff had the opportunity to learn from attending physicians with greater experience and understanding of the challenges involved in treating the individual patient. At the same time, the attending physicians had the opportunity to learn from younger and more recently trained house staff who often had more current information about newer tests, procedures, and pharmaceuticals and their potential benefits and risks. Exploiting these various potential advantages required a "team" approach.

Unfortunately, even when the team was working well (from its point of view), it was often the case that the frustrated patient was unable to determine the hierarchical relations among team members, who—or whether any one person—was "in charge," indeed whether the set of physicians really was a "team." Patients and their families frequently complained that they did not know to which physician to turn and with whom to raise questions of concern. Furthermore, even in those circumstances where a well-functioning team was in place, patients were often tempted to conclude that the various individual physicians, who were specialists and subspecialists, viewed the patient as a collection of organs rather than as a whole person. They did not believe that competent care and compassionate care needed to be mutually exclusive.

As university medical centers grew (and came to house increasingly costly and sophisticated new technology and, one might add, increasingly costly staff) and as private health insurance spread, these centers were transformed from serving mainly low-income uninsured populations, often under conditions that treated these patients as "teaching material" (indeed, that term was frequently used to describe the hospitalized low-income patient),[18] to serving insured, including affluent, patients who required the expertise available in these centers. Rashi Fein remembers well the dean of a great university medical school expressing his misgivings about the expansion of private Blue Cross hospital insurance because, in his view, this would mean that the hospital would no longer have "captive" nonpaying patients whom it could use for "teaching purposes."

Moreover, it was often the case that medical centers had to educate their more affluent fully insured patients that the advantages of the medical center far outweighed whatever "intrusions" occurred because of the presence of medical students and the growing number of house staff. Clearly, they succeeded in convincing their patients that insurance payments were buying good medical care and that was worth the loss of privacy. In fact, it can be said that they were so persuasive that patients preferred the teaching hospital (in spite of its "crisis" atmosphere) even when the required procedure could be performed in a smaller community hospital. This preference of course has been a matter of continuing concern to insurers since the teaching hospital is a more costly locus of care. A number of insurers now require that subscribers pay the differential if they elect to be treated in more expensive (but not medically necessary) facilities.

Efforts were made to structure these various transitions (changes in patient mix, sources of funding, growth of research) in a more orderly fashion. In 1970 a report by the distinguished Carnegie Commission on Higher Education recommended that with the increasing need for more complex diagnostic and therapeutic care, the medical centers should become the "hubs" of health service programs, characterized by a flow of patients from "primary care" sites to centers.[19] It hoped that this regionalization approach would lead to improved care and a rationalization and more orderly distribution of resources. However, the substitution of the term "regionalization" for the term "planning" was insufficient to overcome the general bias against planning. Nor, of course, could even an adroit choice of words deal with the lack of a coherent financing system for services, the inherently competitive nature of the medical care system, even (perhaps, especially) among institutions of higher education, and the problems and turf issues associated with regionalization in urban areas with several medical schools. As with so many publicly and privately sponsored reports, the Commission's recommendations were largely ineffective.[20]

In an attempt to cope with the managerial problems resulting from the growth of university medical centers and their many educational programs (including activities outside the medical school), a pattern emerged that clustered these various activities under the administration of a vice president for health affairs. While in some cases that position was filled by the medical school dean, that arrangement, quite understandably, came under fire from the various other health professions schools and centers within the university. Even so, in general, medical schools continued to be the dominant component of most university health centers, and their national organization, the Association of American Medical Colleges (AAMC), remained the major national voice speaking on behalf of medical school deans. The significance of the AAMC's role in helping to shape health policy endured even after a new national organization, the Association of Academic Health Centers, came into being in 1958. Not only did the AAMC represent the medical school, the largest part of the university academic medical center, but it also provided a national voice for teaching hospitals through its Council on Teaching Hospitals. Indeed, in 1968 the AAMC moved its offices from Chicago to Washington in order to consolidate its influence in Washington, the center of national policy development affecting medical education (including NIH appropriations and other funds for research).[21] This move had an important symbolic aspect. It served as recognition that federal dollars (both the amounts appropriated and the purposes for which they were made available) were vitally important, and that in that sense the locus of financial stability and its corollary, power, lay in the legislative and executive branches of the federal government.

The Expansion of Physician Supply

As research and patient care expanded, educational programs understandably appeared relatively smaller and less central to the mission of the health sciences centers and of the medical schools. Independently, though perhaps influenced by the feeling that the education portion of the three-legged stool (education, research, and service) was out of balance, strong pressures developed to expand the education of physicians (as well as that of other health professions) and to improve its quality. By the 1950s, aided by the accelerated programs of the medical schools during World War II,[22] there had been a return to the immediate pre-Flexnerian levels of numbers (about 5,500) of medical school graduates.[23] But the number of new entrants (the flow) was so small relative to the total number of physicians (the stock) that the supply available to serve a growing population did not increase rapidly. Indeed, the ratio of physicians to population did not return to the levels found at the turn of the century until the late 1970s.[24]

Inevitably, and especially so in a society in which the watchword seemed to be "more is better," there was a growing pressure to expand the capacity of medical schools and, thereby, increase the number of physicians. The pressure was fueled by the aging of the population and consequent increase in needed interventions, by the impact of affluence, which increased the demand for medical care, and by the spread of health insurance that decreased the financial barriers to care. It was also fueled by the desire to increase enrollment of under-represented ethnic, racial, and gender groups (without "taking away" places from white males); by the attitude, common among economists, that increases in the supply of physicians would help moderate the inflation in physician fees; and, finally, by the view that it was far more "dangerous" to have too few physicians than too many (a corollary of the— often incorrect—view that "underdoctoring" is more dangerous than "overdoctoring").[25] Furthermore, the American Medical Association's earlier guild-like and "protectionist" behavior led many to question the view that an expansion in the number of physicians would reduce quality.

Perhaps the most forceful and influential statement on the need for an increased supply of physicians had been found in the report of the Surgeon-General's Consultant Group on Medical Education (the Bane Report) in 1959, which projected the need for 40,000 additional physicians by 1975.[26] At the time there were 236,000 physicians in practice.[27] Although the Group attempted to justify its recommendations, the "methodology" seemed to rely heavily on "expert opinion" and left one with the feeling that there was no precise way of knowing what the appropriate number should be. Public officials often spoke about a need for 40,000 to 50,000 additional physicians.[28] The enactment of Medicare and Medicaid in 1965 led many to believe that demand for physician services would grow and that training more physicians to meet that demand was a national priority. The rapid acceleration in medical care costs after the implementation of these two programs served to validate their prediction. Few asked whether "physician services" needed to be performed by physicians, that is, whether other personnel (such as nurse practitioners or physician assistants) might not substitute for more costly physicians. Few took note of the fact that prepaid group practices functioned with very different ratios of various personnel to subscribers (and with fewer physicians) than was true in the rest of the system.[29]

The national response to the warnings of an emerging crisis in the delivery of care because of an impending physician shortage was dramatic. As early as 1963 it led to the passage of the Health Professions Educational Assistance Act, designed to increase medical school enrollments. The Act and subsequent amendments provided construction funds (on a matching basis) for medical schools, along with per student "capitation funds" conditioned on school commitments to increases in class size. The latter (ranging from $500,000 to $1,000,000 per school) were particularly enticing since they provided deans with discretionary funds, which were always in short supply. Though medical school administrators chafed at the notion that the receipt of federal money would be accompanied by constraints and notions of accountability, these constraints were not burdensome, nor did federal policies require a monolithic response. It therefore was not surprising that in spite of the newly posed obligations, no schools turned down the financial assistance. Loans to students also became available and, ultimately, Congress enacted a federal scholarship program (the National Health Service Corps) with the provision that students repay their scholarships through service in medically underserved areas.[30]

In addition to these federal policy initiatives, many states significantly increased their support for expansion of existing medical schools and provided funds for the establishment of new ones. A number of state legislatures, primarily in states with low physician to population ratios, continued to fund the development of new schools (and did so even during the early 1980s when there already was a growing concern that the United States was developing a surplus of physicians). These legislatures believed that admission policies that gave preference to in-state residents would lead graduates and associated house staff in the teaching hospitals to enter practice in the state and help solve the chronic problem of geographic maldistribution of physicians. They also hoped that these schools, often conceptualized as community-based, with a family practice and/or primary care or rural services orientation, would lead to a new emphasis on the delivery of primary care services to underserved state residents. One school founded in 1973, the Sophie Davis School of Biomedical Education, the medical school of the City University of New York (CUNY), defined its primary mission as graduating physicians to serve the poor, particularly members of minority groups.

Federal and state legislation and appropriations were remarkably effective in increasing the number of schools and the number of graduating physicians. In the two decades from 1960 to 1980, forty-one new allopathic schools of medicine and eight new schools of osteopathic medicine were established. The numbers of graduating medical students more than doubled from 7,500 in 1960 to 16,200 in 1980. Furthermore, it is fair to say that the expansion in admissions helped reduce (though not always eliminate) potential tensions that otherwise might have arisen had it been necessary to reduce white male admissions in order to increase enrollment of minority students and, as well, to expand the enrollment of women who had also faced a long history of discrimination in admission.[31] As is true in many areas of life, medical school admission committees found it easier to reallocate resources when those resources were increasing and when providing additional opportunities to some did not mean decreasing opportunities for others.

Measures to expand enrollment were so successful that by the late 1970s concern developed over a surplus of physicians, and Congress mandated that the Secretary of the Department of Health, Education, and Welfare appoint a Graduate Medical Education National Advisory Committee (GMENAC) to assess future needs for physicians. Its 1980 report projected that the United States would have a surplus of 70,000 physicians by 1990 and 140,000 by the year 2000.[32] These numbers were just as questionable as the earlier ones that had proclaimed shortages since there was little agreement on what adequacy might mean, on the potential impact of HMOs and other organizational and financing changes, or on shifts in medicine's scientific and technical base.

As indicated, any analyses of physician supply and needs would have been difficult given the various uncertainties; this would have been the case even if the United States were an island unto itself. Nonetheless, augmenting the issues already discussed was the substantial increase in the number of graduates of foreign medical schools who were entering medical practice in the United States, and the growing recognition that this situation was likely to continue. During the 1970s more than 40 percent of all physicians licensed were foreign medical graduates (peaking at over 7,000 physicians in 1973). Though these numbers and percentages declined over time, they remained at over 3,000 physicians and around 20 percent of newly licensed physicians in the early 1980s.[33] The United States appeared to be meeting its physician needs (at least in part) by importing physicians who had received their initial training abroad.

Immigration policies facilitated the recruitment of foreign medical school graduates who were in demand by hospitals, especially large urban hospitals, county and municipal institutions, and state mental hospitals. Though many of these were excellent training institutions, they nevertheless tended to have a lower salary structure, more difficult working conditions, and (on occasion) less "prestige." Consequently, they often were unable to fill their house staff "slots" (and in some cases, their budgeted physician positions) with United States graduates. While, for many purposes, house staff physicians may be considered as students, it is also the case that these "students" represent a source of labor. The teaching hospital and the institutions we have referred to could not function without house staff (whose earnings were much less than would have been required to replace them with physicians recruited out of the practicing physician pool). Thus the needs of these various hospitals were clear and pressing. On the other hand, since many of the foreign-educated physicians who received the Educational Commission for Foreign Medical Graduates (ECFMG) certificate were from developing countries (for example, Korea, India, Pakistan, and the Philippines), there was considerable criticism that the prosperous United States was meeting its needs by depleting the resources of medically poorer nations. Nor could this be viewed as a benign matter in which the United States provided training that added to the "human capital" of the developing nations when these trainees returned to their home countries. Many of these physicians remained in the United States after they had completed their residency and specialty training. Furthermore, the priorities of many of those who did return to their countries of origin often reflected their training in the American health care system, a system with needs and resources quite at variance with those of less affluent nations.

Although there were efforts to restrain the numbers of immigrant physicians, such endeavors ran counter to prevailing notions of free immigration. Moreover, as noted, these "trainees" were welcomed by hospitals that had a crying need for physicians. When it proved impossible to inhibit the inflow of persons seeking training (and whom hospitals wanted to hire), the medical educational establishment set up criteria in the form of a qualifying examination by the ECFMG in an attempt to assure basic levels of knowledge as well as language competence.

As time passed, yet another significant development compounded the problem of estimating the balance between the need for and the supply of physicians. A growing number of United States citizens enrolled in and graduated from foreign medical schools. While there had always been a small number of Americans who attended traditional schools of medicine abroad, an increasing number were enrolling in newly established schools (mainly in the Caribbean area, hence the designation "off-shore" medical schools). These largely for-profit schools were generally regarded as of questionable quality. Nevertheless, they were accredited by the countries in which they were located and therefore were listed by the World Health Organization (WHO) as accredited medical schools. As a consequence they provided the many students turned down by American medical schools (some of whom had been rejected because of the shortage of available spaces rather than because they did not have the qualifications to become able physicians) an opportunity for a medical education in an "approved" school.

Thus the Flexner goal of achieving high quality in medical education through high admission standards, which led to the elimination of proprietary medical schools and to the limitation of the number of places in American medical schools, inadvertently created conditions resulting in a proliferation of proprietary medical schools abroad catering to United States citizens who had strong aspirations to become physicians. The severe restrictions on admissions inspired the development of alternative paths to satisfy needs. The lesson perhaps is that "rationing" needs persuasive justification and acceptance. When these were not forthcoming, escape valves in the form of proprietary off-shore medical schools developed.

Medical educators generally were dismayed by their perception of the (presumed) lower standards that off-shore graduates would bring to medicine, and undoubtedly expected widespread support for their attempt to restrict entry in an effort, as they saw it, to maintain quality and protect the public. They failed to anticipate the political support the families of these students would generate or that this family support would be combined with advocacy by many hospitals that were eager to fill house staff positions. Instead, medical educators were forced to institute various programs designed to accommodate the aspirations of these students, their families, and the needs of hospitals.

The policy of restricting admissions to United States medical schools could be defended if it were the case that those not admitted were individuals who, if admitted, would not have graduated. While this was undoubtedly true in some cases, there was little evidence that it was generally true. After all, some applicants who were not admitted had been placed on a waiting list and thus were deemed admissible. They did not enroll because no vacancy developed. It is interesting to note that the "quality" argument was sometimes presented not as a commentary on applicants, but in reference to how many students the faculty could handle and to the "shortage" of an associated infrastructure such as laboratories and places for microscopes. If nothing else, these arguments underscored the ingenuity (and small-mindedness) of those who controlled the admissions processes.[34] In truth, the number admitted was the result of decisions by individual schools (and state legislatures) who determined the particular school's capacity, and by a federal attempt, using a rough "manpower" model, to react (at the margins) to the balance between the estimates of physician supply and needs. The United States rejected the notion that medical schools should be open to all who had the ability to pursue that course of study. Our approach stood in contrast to the admission policies in many other nations where "open enrollment" prevailed, that is, where the number of medical school places reflected the number of persons who wanted to attend and had the ability to pursue that line of studies successfully.

In no small measure, though full of "loopholes," the manpower approach that tried to balance supply and demand (and in so doing limit the number of physicians) grew out of a concern with high and ever-increasing medical care expenditures. While other nations (with universal coverage) used national budgetary techniques to limit national health expenditures, the United States hoped to intervene, at least in part, by attempting to restrict the growth of resources. The older argument that an increase in the number of physicians would increase competition, and thus restrain price increases for physicians' services and *reduce* expenditures on medical care, was replaced by a newer argument that each additional physician generated more visits, procedures, interventions, hospital admissions, and pharmaceutical prescriptions, and thus would *increase* expenditures. Since each additional physician (presumably) would add some hundreds of thousands of dollars of expenditures to the medical care system, limiting the supply of physicians (presumably) would control the level of total health care expenditures (even if it did increase the price or "cost" of various procedures). Of course, the goal of a health care system is not simply to minimize expenditures. This can be done by having no physicians and providing no care. The goal of the system is to meet the health care needs of the population while not wasting resources or providing "unnecessary" care. That goal did not automatically translate into restrictions on the supply of physicians or the services they provided.

Interestingly, the observation that more doctors would mean more services and would be deleterious to the nation's fiscal health was a variant of the argument that had been used for decades against fee-for-service medicine. A similar argument has been made about the hospital sector in Roemer's law, "a bed built is a bed filled." The equivalent was assumed in the case of physicians. One might have coined a new law: "an M.D. degree granted means health care expenditures expanded." Though the case for limits was often argued on "quality" grounds, limiting the number of physicians became an economic imperative.[35]

Medical Education: Issues of Quality

The rapid expansion in research funding and the growth of research manpower and facilities led to an equally rapid expansion of academic health centers. As already noted, these resulted in chronic expressions

(and not only by students) of anxiety about medical student education. There seemed to be an assumption that a "zero-sum" game was
at work in which an expansion of one leg of the three-legged stool
necessarily came at the expense of one or both of the other legs. These
concerns led to much experimentation with the curriculum and teaching methods. The demonstration at the Case-Western Medical School
that the quality of education did not suffer with a "new" curriculum
(adopted in 1952),[36] and the interest generated by the thirteen annual teaching institutes sponsored by the AAMC in the fifties and sixties, spawned a sense of confidence that flexibility in the curriculum
and teaching methods would assure the maintenance of quality even
in the face of competing research pressures. The prediction by Paul
Sanazaro, the head of the HEW Center for Health Services Research
and Development, that medical schools would become analogous to
liberal arts colleges, requiring some courses but permitting a number
of electives, came to pass.[37] The establishment of many departments or
divisions of medical education indicated that teaching was a matter of
deep concern and not as neglected as was often suggested.[38]

Many reservations were expressed about the length of the educational program and its consequent costs. Allowing for internship and
residency, medical students did not enter practice until they were
some twelve years beyond high school graduation and had incurred
considerable debt. The Institute of Medicine reported that in 1980 over
three-quarters of medical students graduated medical school in debt,
with an average indebtedness at graduation totaling $17,200.[39] Fur-
thermore, both the percentage of students graduating with debts and
the average indebtedness were increasing. Some educators argued that
the prospect of large indebtedness narrowed the base from which
medical students might be drawn and thus the socioeconomic characteristics of the student body.[40] Furthermore, many analysts suggested
that levels of indebtedness influenced selection of a specialty, choice of
a practice location, and fee structures. Nevertheless, there were few
pressures (at least from educators) to shorten the length of training.
Instead, medical educators concentrated their attention on curricular
changes and on the quality of instruction and methods to improve it.

The curricular changes that did develop were quite eclectic. As biomedical research moved increasingly toward molecular biology, the disciplinary boundaries of the basic sciences became less distinct. For example, as microbiology lent itself to new methods of the study of genetics, it became more like biochemistry. As a consequence there were many curricular efforts to introduce or strengthen interdisciplinary teaching programs in the basic sciences. Other efforts were directed at "vertical integration," that is, bringing some or more clinical teaching into the student's experience in the first two years. These inspired (sometimes successful) attempts to reorganize the departmental structure of the medical school. Still other efforts were directed at increasing the student's understanding of human development. This often took the form of adding an introductory course in psychiatry or the "behavioral sciences" in the first two years of the curriculum. This approach was manifested by greater attention to the teaching of the doctor-patient relationship.[41] These innovations were conceptualized by George L. Engel of the University of Rochester as the biopsychosocial teaching of medicine.[42]

None of these developments were carried forward in isolation. As early as 1969 McMaster Medical School in Hamilton, Ontario, had fundamentally altered its approach to medical education and had adopted a "problem-based" curriculum.[43] This new teaching program presented clinical cases, the "problems," and expected students to learn on their own (though ultimately together with other students and faculty) by "addressing" these problems. This curriculum received a great deal of attention, and it and other curricular reforms were part of a continuing and healthy ferment. Some educators suggested (perhaps counting on a "placebo" or "Hawthorne" effect) that every curriculum needed changing after a decade or so.

In 1981 the then-dean at the Harvard Medical School introduced a comprehensive reform called the "New Pathway." Among other transformations, such as dividing the entering class into smaller groupings called "societies," time spent listening to lectures was substantially reduced. Instead, based to a significant degree on the McMaster model, the curriculum recognized that, in general, students were coming into medical school with much more preparation in the sciences than had been true in earlier periods, and that it therefore was possible and desirable to teach the basic sciences around and in the context of clinical case problems. The "New Pathway" also enabled earlier clinical exercises, greater emphasis on the doctor-patient relationship, and extensive use of computer simulations of laboratory exercises.[44] Of course, other medical schools also adopted curricular changes, but since, as at Harvard, medical schools introduced many changes simultaneously, it was difficult, if not impossible, to assess the impact of each of the various innovations. Schools did not know which of the many modifications made by a sister school was of higher priority and worth copying. Such information would have been useful even if each school exercised its freedom (one of the strengths of American higher education) and met its need for change in its own way, based on its own history, conditions, and resources.

Students who entered medical schools not only had better preparation in the basic sciences; they were also more knowledgeable about computers and their various applications. While the desktop computer had not become ubiquitous by the mid-1980s, it was clear that we were very close to incorporating the digital revolution into the educational environment. An increasing proportion of hospitals (and physicians) began shifting to the use of electronic records in clinical settings. It would not be long before we would witness the emergence of communication by e-mail, publication of electronic journals and books, the possibility of doing library research at one's desk via the Internet, and creation of computer-generated three-dimensional representations of the human body and of laboratory-designed drugs. The extensive use of computers and the revolution in telecommunications (which rendered much amphitheatre-type teaching unnecessary, if not obsolete) forced a reshaping of the physical setting of the medical schools. These various developments had the desirable effect of focusing attention on the educational programs and on computer-assisted learning.

While some innovative programs worked and others did not, it is important to note that, in general, medical educators recognized that the medical school had to adjust to changes in the student body, in medicine's knowledge base, as well as in available technologies, and that experimentation and reevaluation were necessary. Again, as with the basic curriculum, different schools tried different approaches, ones that seemed to suit their faculties, students, and special conditions. Outside observers could express skepticism about the amount of time, energy, and money that was allocated to "self-study," to "strategic planning," and to the implementation of ideas that various reports proposed. What they failed to consider was that this ferment offered evidence that medical schools were not fossilized. They were very much alive in trying to acclimate to a large number of alterations in their internal and external environments.

In a paradoxical way the anxiety over the displacement of teaching by the growth of research seemed to have the effect of keeping educational commitment very much alive and front and center. To some outside observers the rise in numbers of faculty members and the expansion of physical facilities appeared to offer evidence that the students' educational experiences were becoming increasingly fragmented. Nevertheless, the quality of the newly minted physicians did not appear to suffer. Curricula and teaching methods became more varied, but there is no evidence that results, as judged by test performance and preparation for further clinical training, declined. One should not discount the ability and resilience of medical students or the commitment of some faculty members to making the system work even in the face of impediments caused by rapid advances, fragmentation, and shifting priorities.

The difficulties that the health sector faced were real. So, too, was the unhappiness of many patients in their interactions and encounters with the world of medicine (and with physicians who, after all, were often the patient's entrée to that world). It was tempting to believe that if "things weren't right," say, in the patient-doctor relationship, there was something wrong with medical education. Yet patient unhappiness was more often related to system problems involving organization and financing issues than to inadequate physician training and matters of technical competence. We do not imply that all medical schools and educators gave sufficient priority to the importance of sensitizing their students to the needs that patients would have in their encounters with individual physicians and with the medical care system. Indeed, far too often medical students were ignorant of financing and organization issues, had little understanding of the health care system, and lacked the experience and ability to see things from the patient's perspective. Nor do we imply that physicians who were curt and abrupt and who failed to communicate effectively with their patients exhibited these behavioral characteristics solely because of increased emphasis on research or technology or because of hectic time pressures.

Dr. Fein recalls that already in the early 1950s, well before the spread of technological marvels and well before physicians were "harassed" by the need to fill out countless forms, his question about the number of treatments that he might need for a particular condition was answered by the consulting physician in a memorable way: "If you wanted to know that, why didn't you go to medical school?" All of us are well aware that concerned and frightened patients seek help (care in addition to cure), and that help is not always forthcoming. It is certainly the case that many educators were aware that physicians did not always exhibit the compassion that some patients sought. One would have to have led an extremely cloistered life to be ignorant that this was a common patient (or family) complaint. Undoubtedly, some medical educators felt that they did not know how to teach "compassion." There surely were others who believed that compassion was that "soft" stuff that could easily be summed up as "being nice," something that need not take curriculum time away from basic science and clinical care. Yet we are aware that was not a dominant view: many medical educators were trying to develop curricula that valued the patient as a person and to do so even in the face of competing priorities such as generating research dollars and patient fees. In fact, many educators felt that because of research and service pressures, such curricular materials (as with bioethical issues) were increasingly necessary.

The institutionalization of house staff training following World War II and its prolongation to four years (and longer if subspecialization were pursued) undoubtedly facilitated the experimentation with curricula for the medical student. Faculty members knew that the four years of medical school did not represent the terminal education, as had usually been the case prior to World War II when additional training most often consisted of a one-year internship. Faculties understood that they had to examine the impact of these changes on their curricula. Importantly, at the same time, they could be more relaxed about considering and adopting variation in teaching. Residency training provided a valued safety net.

As curricular changes permitted individual medical schools to become somewhat more differentiated from each other, a school's history and tradition, along with current statements of mission, helped to define the "character" of a school. At the extremes some schools regarded themselves (and were regarded by others) as being primarily interested in graduating students who would pursue research careers while others emphasized graduating students for primary care practice. Nevertheless, graduates from the research-oriented schools often ended up in clinical practice, and those of primary care-oriented schools often became subspecialists. Thus every school had to have underlying breadth and strength.

It is worth noting that many critics of the drift toward specialization thought that specialist medical school faculty members (who often had national reputations and were leaders in their specialty societies) diverted students from careers in primary care, if only by example and as role models. This was seldom the case. Important as the examples of individual faculty members may have been, they probably were secondary to the students' observations about developments in medicine. Students were aware of the trend toward specialization and subspecialization and deemed it inevitable. Many (though not all) wanted to participate in what they saw as expanding practice opportunities and reap the associated economic rewards (all the more so, given the debt burdens they assumed).

Studies of primary care indicated that by and large student background and characteristics, rather than medical school experience, determined the selection of a career in primary care, and especially so in the choice to practice in a rural area. In recent years there is mounting evidence that an increasing proportion of students consider "lifestyle" issues—personal free time and total weekly hours spent on work responsibilities—when they select a specialty.[45] Medical school admissions committees could take such factors into account if they placed a sufficiently high priority on increasing the number of persons enter-

ing primary care or family practice. The variations in choice of practice among graduates of American medical schools in fact suggest that
schools do have (and have acted upon) different priorities.[46]

State licensure and/or a passing performance on part I and II of the
examinations sponsored by the National Board of Medical Examiners
provide the basic legal entitlement to practice medicine. By the 1960s,
however, most physicians went on to specialty board certification
(training for family practice became a specialty with residency training requirements in 1969). In that sense quality standards in medical
training (including residency training) and of medical practice were directly and indirectly under the jurisdiction of the medical specialty
boards. Despite the diversity of settings in which training took place,
the accreditation process for residency training programs was sufficiently careful to assure the competence of practitioners who passed
the qualifying examinations.

Nevertheless, there was a growing concern about the wide variation across the United States in practice modalities, number of procedures, length of hospital stay, and so forth. As indicated, students of
medical care issues had long been aware that these kinds of variations
were often found between fee-for-service and prepaid group practice
(later HMO) medicine. The newer studies indicated that such variations were also present between similar practice modalities.[47] Since the
variations were quite wide and could not be explained by severity of
illness or patient characteristics, there were substantial grounds for
concern. It was apparent that not every practitioner could be doing the
right thing!

Either some patients were receiving less care than appropriate or, alternatively, some patients were receiving more care than appropriate
(or both). These differences had important implications for quality of
care and risk. They also had substantial cost consequences. Considerable effort was expended to ascertain the basis for these variations. The
easy (but as it turned out, incorrect) assumption was that the differences reflected the educational experience in medical school and/or
the training experience associated with particular hospitals. Nevertheless, though these factors may have exerted marginal influence, the
wide differences appeared to result from geographic factors, includ-

ing the availability of resources in the medical "market" in which the physician practiced and accepted prevailing medical practices in that market.[48]

As a consequence the studies of these variations, important as they were in understanding medical practice, had little impact on the education and training in medical schools and their affiliated hospitals— beyond the important lesson that prevailing practice could (and should) be questioned. Medical educators and administrators surely were relieved to conclude that the solution to the important issues raised by these variations lay outside their domain and responsibility. Of course, observers could ask a reasonable question: if the effort to reduce variation was not the responsibility of medical education, then in whose domain did the search for a solution lie? Indeed, to whom should the question be addressed?

Although the debates about the intake capacity of medical schools were dominated by a manpower or labor need and supply model, and even though an increasing proportion of physicians were trained and practiced as specialists, the numbers of specialists trained and their distribution among the various specialties bore no or little relationship to the projected needs of the population. The approach to these supply issues was quite inconsistent. The attempts at specificity in planning aspects of total physician supply, as if physicians were homogeneous, stood in sharp contrast to the fewer and weaker efforts concerning the far more important issue of the supply of physicians by specialty. The numbers trained in each specialty and subspecialty evolved eclectically from the number of residents in each training center, which in turn was determined by the number that respective chiefs of services thought necessary or desirable to provide clinical care in that institution. Since residents represented relatively cheap labor, there typically were more residencies available than could be filled by United States medical graduates. As already noted, foreign medical graduates filled this gap.

During the periods of rapid growth in facilities and health expenditures in the decades of the fifties, sixties, and seventies, training programs that were producing large numbers of specialists did not appear to pose a problem. All trainees found opportunities to practice medicine. Ultimately, however, the graduates of these approved training programs could not all be absorbed in academic training centers. The newly minted specialists began to develop autonomous specialized centers to compete with the very institutions in which they had trained. Chiefs of services of training programs who felt they needed the trainees in order to fill service needs were increasingly concerned about what happened to their trainees later and whether the quality of their practices outside of medical centers would be sufficiently high. They also wondered whether the supply of patients would be large enough to enable their own academic centers to maintain their patient loads and, thus, their training programs in the face of the "competitors" whom they were training. Observers of the emerging competition wondered whether this "oversupply" of specialists would not inevitably induce an increase in health care interventions and associated costs even as it reduced the average quality of practice.[49] Or, mindful of the rising number of specialists, these same onlookers might be puzzled by United States policies that tried to address concerns about the level of health expenditures and, at the same time, encouraged the expansion in the supply of resources.

Thus concern about an impending surplus of specialists was added to the national concern about a surplus of medical school graduates. One could imagine that eventually market forces and changes in relative incomes of various specialties might play a role in "curing" the allocation problem, but there was agreement that, at best, the corrective and feedback mechanisms would take a long time before they had the necessary impact. One could look forward to an expansion of HMOs, expecting that they would exert control over the number of procedures they would approve and, consequently, over the number of physicians with whom they would associate, but that day had not yet come. The American dilemma, on the one hand, of wanting to rely on market forces yet nevertheless being skeptical about their efficacy, and, on the other hand, wanting something akin to the results of rational planning while rejecting planners and planning mechanisms—that is, the dilemma of wanting lower expenditures while rejecting control and budgeting mechanisms—shaped how we dealt, and did not deal, with graduate medical education. There were symposia, conferences, reports, and recommendations, but the medical community was not yet ready to break with the old traditional view that, unlike other occupations and professions, physicians were free to decide what to practice, where to practice, and on whom to practice, that is, that physicians did not face an employment market.

While the medical community did not intervene in the allocation of residency positions (and therefore in the number of practitioners in the various specialties), it felt comfortable in addressing traditional quality issues. Spurred by the growing consumer movement of the sixties and the increasing complexity of medical knowledge and practice, leaders in both the medical community and government sought to assure that practitioners remained competent after licensure and certification. The specialty boards developed programs for recertification through examinations (usually at three-year intervals). In addition, various states instituted requirements that practitioners enroll in and attend a specified number of hours of course work per year. This resulted in the emergence of a cottage industry in continuing medical education courses, often under the auspices of academic medical centers. At a time when practitioners were feeling ever more harassed by regulations and paper work required by insurers and government reimbursing agencies, the documentation of attendance was regarded as onerous, but physicians had to comply.

It is important and troubling to note that many of the continuing medical education courses were sponsored, at least in part, by pharmaceutical firms (and were sometimes held in luxurious vacation settings) with attendance paid for in whole or in substantial part by those same companies. It was clear that these "informational" sessions were of value to the sponsors in exerting subtle and not so subtle influences on prescribing practice. Thus those arrangements, which undoubtedly removed some of the physician opposition to the imposition of "requirements," raised and continue to raise numerous conflict-of-interest issues.[50]

These continuing medical education and recertification efforts, designed to assure that practitioners maintained their skills, were well intentioned. Nevertheless, they could not be more than proxies for clinical performance. Although "audits" of office practice became a component of some recertification programs, there was no agreed-upon acceptable way to judge how well a physician performed in a day-to-day clinical setting. Regrettably, informal peer review also did not serve well. The threat of litigation led physicians, hospital administrators, and medical societies to keep information about performance quiet. Dr. Fein recalls asking some hundreds of members of a state medical society whether they knew any physicians whom they felt their own family members should avoid. The overwhelming majority responded in the affirmative. Nevertheless, when asked why they were unwilling to "do something about it" in order to protect the public at large and in order to avoid government intervention and handle the problem "within the family," the president of the society intervened with a reminder that if they attempted to deal with "incompetence in some formal manner," they would have to face the threat of suit. In turn, that would require an increase in dues. It became clear that these physicians would readily advise their family members on aspects of physician competence, but were disinclined to take action that would protect all patients. Though refusing to act through their society, they nevertheless continued to decry government attempts to police the system—particularly through licensure—in an effort to improve quality.[51]

An Overview

It would have been easy to conclude that the "educational establishment" had made remarkable progress in the decades that spanned the later sixties, seventies, and early 1980s. In large measure this was true. The period under discussion began with student protests, but, painful as those years were, they led to changes that brought important benefits to the medical schools and schools of public health. The shift in the relationships between students and faculty from very hierarchal to (somewhat) collegial, and the growth (as a consequence of expansion of enrollment) in the number of faculty, which in turn influenced the gender distribution (and to a lesser extent the racial and ethnic distribution) of faculty, enriched the institutions and the students' experiences. The transformation in the composition of the student body helped make the schools a more integral part of the society and raised the prospect that graduates would alter the geographic distribution of practitioners and the areas of specialization.

It was also the case that medical schools and schools of public health had gone through a period of great expansion—there were more of them, and the schools themselves were larger—and had done remarkably well in adjusting to those changes in scale. Deans of other faculties in the university undoubtedly were envious of what to the outsider appeared to be the medical school's embarrassment of riches, which enabled an academic style of life (secretarial and technical assistance, books, supplies, and travel) far different than that of the prevailing image of the penurious professor, and certainly different than prevailing standards in many other departments in the university. Of course, not every medical school was well endowed, not every school could count on affluent donors, and not every school was successful in attracting research funds. Yet it is fair to say that, in general, medical schools were among the more affluent divisions in their parent universities. Indeed, some of the tensions that medical schools faced were related to their relative affluence and to the attempts by various university presidents to use funds that the medical schools felt were theirs to help subsidize other parts of the collective educational enterprise. The "wealthy relative" often was more resented than admired.

Another internal tension could be found between the medical school and its faculty on the one hand and its teaching hospital on the other. In some schools the hospital was the dominant (and domineering) partner and its fiscal problems became the concern of the medical school faculty and, depending on the fiscal arrangements between the school and hospital and consequent impact on the school faculty, of the medical school administration. Hospital directors and vice presidents for finance were aware that medical students slowed things down and added to costs. They knew that medical faculty members wanted more and more research space and less and less contact with patients. Dr. Fein remembers a professor in graduate school declaring that "this wouldn't be a bad job if it weren't for the students." It is not an exaggeration to suggest that some teaching hospital administrators similarly felt that they would get along well with their medical school counterparts if only the medical school could get rid of both its faculty and students. It was curious that, as part of the university, the medical school was to be envied, and yet, as part of the division of health affairs, it sometimes found that, relative to the teaching hospital, it was a mere, and somewhat unpopular, appendage.

Nevertheless, by and large it was a good time for the medical school, its faculty, and students. The schools were lively beehives of research activity, much of which was truly exciting basic science with the potential to contribute to progress in health. Further, busy as senior and junior faculty were, most schools had an ethos that placed great value on "mentoring," which served to socialize students and foster collegiality. It is striking how many students have fond memories of particular professors, how many faculty members remember their students, and how often student-faculty member associations blossomed into relationships that spanned decades. Undoubtedly, the close ties that were forged also stimulated the periodic (and frequent) attempts to strengthen the curriculum and to improve teaching performance.

Of course, there were nagging problems. Student debt levels were increasing, and both students and faculty were aware and troubled that economic factors were intruding on personal decisions about such matters as specialization, location of practice, and allocation of time. Conflict-of-interest issues were more frequent as well as more complex and troublesome. The polarization in the greater society (on such matters as abortion) found its counterparts (although more muted) in the university. Yet the medical school could feel that it was "special." It was far too close to the real world and its problems to be considered an ivory tower, but those who were within its walls could feel somehow protected from many of the issues about health care agitating the outside world. Those were the difficult medical care access and delivery issues that medical school faculty believed, quite incorrectly, would affect them only at the margin.

For a number of reasons the mutations in the world of medical care were not a matter of intense analytic discussion in faculty or departmental meetings. Certainly, participants were as confused by the various transformations as were most citizens. Yet the fact that they were expert clinicians and/or imaginative and persevering scientists did not equip them for debates about the future of health care, nor had their earlier education done so. Furthermore, they were already fully engaged and trying to understand and stay current with the new scientific knowledge and new clinical procedures. Like most of us, they expressed their irritations about a host of matters, including the state of health care, but (again, like most of us) they were aware that being confused, irritated, and even angry is not synonymous with feeling one knows what to do about the problem, that one has command of one's future. It was as if they were officers on a ship, officers who did not know who was in charge (or, indeed, whether anyone was) or where the ship was heading. They recognized that fundamental changes were taking place, suspected that even more would take place in the future, and feared that the various changes would be for the worse. In our judgment they were correct in all three conclusions.

The medical care system, having addressed some of the issues it faced in developing means to improve access to care, had tried to deal with the rise in health care expenditures through regulation. But regulation was found wanting, in no small measure because it proceeded on an ad hoc basis and did not deal with the gross inefficiencies and administrative costs of a highly competitive insurance sector. Nor did it effectively attempt to constrain the continuing expansion of resources and proliferation of technology since it remained wedded to a "deficit" model and, on occasion, associated an increase in "supply" with a decline in prices while forgetting that could (and did) lead to an increase in expenditures. Policy makers were torn between two approaches that could not be reconciled: (1) greater health expenditures, deplored as evidence of a misallocation of national resources, did not lead to greater health or better outcomes; (2) greater health expenditures, welcomed as a reflection of our ability and aspiration to do more for more people, were the desirable end result of the advances in science and in clinical care.

As often happens with such conflicting choices, the response was to adopt both points of view. In health care we continued to regulate (ineffectively and by attempting to constrain demand) and to increase resources (and expand supply and expenditures). When forced to choose, public policy avoided choice. Instead, it selected the market as the ultimate arbiter. The impersonal market, presumably reflecting the wants, needs, and desires of (presumably) all the population, would determine the "correct" outcome. But the market perspective of "one dollar, one vote" was at variance with the doctrine of "one person, one vote." In ignoring the distribution of income, it ignored the fact that some individuals have many more votes than others.

The reliance on market forces and the rapid growth of dollars in the health care system proved to be an invitation to the emergence of health care entrepreneurs. We were about to embark on an entrepreneurial revolution that health professionals could not have imagined or dreamed of just two decades earlier.

Part III

MOVING TO THE PRESENT
(1985–2005)

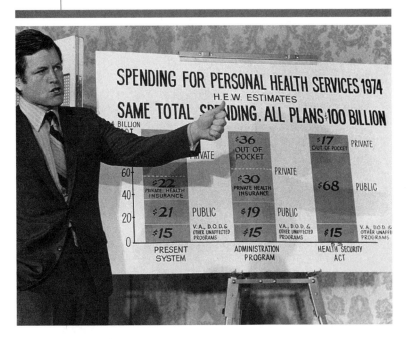

Senator Edward Kennedy explains his and President Nixon's national health insurance proposals in 1974. Neither program was enacted, and the next major NHI debate did not occur until twenty years later under President Clinton. Photograph © CORBIS.

5 | The Entrepreneurial Revolution: A Changing Face for Medicine

It is understandable that when, as at the end of World War II, health expenditures were approximately 4.5 percent of GDP, investors and financiers had little interest in the health sector. But by the mid-1980s, as national health expenditures increased to over $400 billion and almost 11 percent of the GDP, financiers saw the delivery of health care services as a significant part of the American economy and an area for potential investment and possible profit. The interest in health delivery organizations that generated profits was not an entirely new development: for-profit hospitals had long existed, mainly in the southern and southwest United States. Nevertheless, even excluding municipal, county, state, and federal hospitals, the United States health care delivery sector was dominated by not-for-profit institutions.

Growing Expenditures, Increasing Complexity, and the Rise of For-Profits

Although, in time, for-profit HMOs would also attract attention on Wall Street, the move to for-profit organizations began with hospitals. This is not surprising since hospital care constituted almost 40 percent of total health expenditures and offered significant growth opportunities. The number of for-profit hospitals began to rise and spread into the various regions of the country as early as the 1970s.[1] Since many of these newly sponsored for-profit hospitals were part of expanding corporate for-profit chains, there was an important shift away from local control and community involvement and financial support to a distant corporate headquarters and more centralized loci of control. We became familiar with such names as Hospital Corporation of America, Humana, and Tenet.

Furthermore, the aging of the population and the presence of Medicaid funding for long-term care led to the expansion of the nursing-home sector.[2] This expansion required the investment of capital (which was not as readily available to not-for-profits on a loan basis). In turn, this led to an increase in the proportion of for-profit nursing homes and for-profit chains and the growth of yet another politically powerful group that favored additional commercial inroads into the health sector.

Concomitant with the growth of these for-profit sectors was the corporatization of much of medical practice. In retrospect it is surprising that the medical profession did not offer significant resistance to this trend. Part of the explanation lay in the fact that the largest organization of physicians, the American Medical Association (AMA), had long opposed any systematic planning for the delivery of medical care services. Consequently, financial flows and organizational arrangements were left to the marketplace. Physicians were now reaping what AMA ideology had sown.

The irony was that organized medicine in the form of the AMA had focused its attention on government as the threat to physician independence, power, and control, and did not recognize that the marketplace and the behavior of employers who were large purchasers of insurance and of investors who were "medical care entrepreneurs" would represent an even larger threat. While organized medicine could lobby government, it could not identify a locus for exerting pressure against employers who were more actively questioning the costs of and expenditures for medical care. Nor could it identify a locus for resisting the forces of Wall Street that were seeking new opportunities to increase profits by constraining physician behavior and cutting costs. Organized medicine knew where and when the legislature was meeting in open session; it was unable to find its way to closed boardroom doors. The failure to provide adequate representation for America's physicians did not enhance the AMA's status within the profession.

New professional organizations that reflected the increase in specialization and subspecialization were similarly unable to oppose the for-profit developments.[3] As noted, these specialty organizations had their own agendas and interests. Though their leadership tended to be more professionally prestigious than was true for the AMA and usually included faculty members from academic health science centers,[4] they too were ill prepared to address such questions as the structure of American medicine or its place in the larger society. Safe in their class-rooms and their laboratories and protected in their clinical settings by their hospitals, they believed they were insulated from market forces. Those who practiced in teaching hospitals had set up new practice plans to accommodate Medicare and Medicaid legislation. The consultants and financial managers who assisted them were not equipped to address broader health policy issues. So it was that academic physicians devoted their energies to professional matters, which, in their opinion, did not include the way care could be organized and financed. It would be much later that concern with those issues would rise to the surface. As a consequence of the decline in stature and relevance of the AMA and the inability of the specialty societies to fill the public policy vacuum, there was a marked weakening of medicine's influence and power.[5]

It is important to note that not all physicians were oblivious or opposed to the growth of the corporatization of medical practice and the increase in potential profit. After all, Americans value markets (even if we do not entirely trust them) and respect their performance as an allocative device (even if on occasion with ambivalence). There were many who felt that important health sector problems stemmed from shielding health care institutions from market forces. They felt that without the market discipline (presumably) found in the rest of the economy or at least in the for-profit segment, health care would continue to be grossly inefficient and inordinately expensive. That there were physicians who looked upon for-profit hospitals with favor should come as no surprise. What was significant was that, among some, these attitudes had operational consequences. A number of individuals changed or blurred their professional roles as physicians and became important, and on occasion successful, executive and managerial figures in for-profit health care enterprises. Though they held the

Doctor of Medicine degree, it is questionable whether they all could be considered "physicians" since, in some (though, we hasten to add, not all) cases, they had never practiced medicine and could not bring that range of experience to their role as corporate officers. The medical degree may have been irrelevant, but it conferred prestige and status.

Whether or not they had practiced medicine, these physicians faced conflicts of interest between their presumed roles as physicians and their actual roles as corporate managers. These conflicts arose most frequently in the context of the managerial decision to constrain clinical decision making by medical practitioners. At the same time that the executives' loyalty to the organization, to its shareholders, and to its goal of profit maximization called for tighter and tighter controls on the physicians whom they employed or reimbursed, their loyalty to medicine and its ethos called for greater clinical freedom for the practitioner. Since these doctor/managers (often young, energetic, in command of the language of economics and business, and viewed as "the wave of the future") were active in medical organizations, they served to attenuate medically-led opposition to ongoing corporatization.

The change in the physician's role was reflected in the growth in the number of medical students and physicians who enrolled in schools of business administration (often in pursuit of a degree as Master of Business Administration, the MBA) and who in the past might have enrolled in schools of public health. The number of MD/MBA programs exploded from six in 1993 to thirty-three in 2001. Furthermore, by 2003 some seventeen additional schools were considering similar programs.[6] An important byproduct of this development was the increased attention that business school faculty and students accorded developments in the health sector. Faculty who previously had looked askance at or had little interest in trying to apply their methodologies to the not-for-profit health sector noted the development of for-profit institutions and the growth of not-for-profits (sometimes, through mergers or acquisitions) and were intrigued with the health sector's size, characteristics, and performance.

Even the language of medicine changed; the new vocabulary spoke of competition, producers, consumers, and profit centers. Already in 1982 the *New England Journal of Medicine* published a "Sounding

Board" article entitled "What Is Wrong with the Language of Medicine," which discussed the new language of the commercial marketplace that was influencing the discourse in medicine. In this "new language" patients had become customers and physicians had become providers.[7] A decade later a *Journal* editor expressed concern that "we ourselves are confused about what we are. At two extremes we are either a profession or a business; in fact, we are a little of each. We started out as a profession, dedicated, as Hippocrates said, to entering 'every house where I come . . . only for the good of my patients.' The change from personal payment for services to payment by third parties, the decline of voluntarism, and the notion, fostered by government programs such as Medicare, of a payment for each rendered medical service all contributed to the shift toward a marketplace mentality. Whether intentionally or not, many have tilted toward the business end of the spectrum."[8]

The rise in public and private third-party reimbursements for health services greatly facilitated the corporatization of medical practice along with what some referred to as the proletarianization of the medical profession.[9] The AMA's historic defense of fee-for-service (FFS) practice withered away under the pressure of market forces as an increasing number of physicians (including many who remained in independent practice and in a technical sense were not "employees") became partially or totally dependent on salary, capitation, or other contracted income arrangements.

These new and different compensation arrangements had been an expressed goal of those who had looked to not-for-profit, community-oriented, prepaid group practice (PGP) as a desirable organizational pattern for the American medical delivery system. They had long argued that fee-for-service medicine generated "overdoctoring." While it was true that salary and capitated arrangements could generate "underdoctoring," the proponents of PGPs felt they were protected from that outcome by the traditional medical ethos, by the fact that in the typical PGP physicians practiced together and thus in a sense were looking over each other's shoulders, and, importantly, by the not-for-profit environment in which physicians served the needs of their patients.

As for-profit, capitated, prepayment HMOs developed, the environment and analytic models changed. The newer salary and other contractual arrangements (often including bonuses for restraining utilization, most especially of hospital days, but also of costly diagnostic procedures) were part and parcel of an entrepreneurial approach that stressed profits and economic performance rather than quality and patient needs. It could be argued that if quality depreciated, subscribers would leave. Undoubtedly this might be the case in extreme situations. Nevertheless, quality could slip a considerable distance before patients would recognize what was happening. Furthermore, the "exit" alternative was not available to those subscribers who were locked into a particular HMO because their employer offered only one enrollment option. That was frequently the case as employers often found that they could negotiate a lower premium if they "delivered" all their employees. Of course, the fact that employers who extolled competition behaved noncompetitively was not an entirely new phenomenon.

In these various contexts the new salary and compensation arrangements could impinge on quality without effective subscriber resistance. The shift from independent practitioner to "employee" or "quasi-employee" status (at least as regards compensation) further marginalized the influence of the medical profession. The lack of a positive program from within the profession was a source of unhappiness and restlessness among some physicians. This manifested itself in alienation, a feeling of impotence, other evidence of malaise and unhappiness, and recurrent calls for "unionization."

Physicians employed by HMOs and hospitals have long had a federal right to unionize. Conversely, under the Sherman Antitrust Act physicians in independent practice historically have not been allowed to do so. The Federal Trade Commission (FTC) has viewed collective negotiations by independent physicians as price-fixing and therefore illegal. In 1996 the Department of Justice and the FTC created a few "antitrust safety zones," specific circumstances in which physicians might collectively negotiate fees with a managed care plan without being subject to prosecution for price-fixing.

In more recent years there have been attempts to enact federal legislation to provide an exemption for nearly all independent physicians to negotiate collectively with managed care plans. Additionally, a number of states have attempted to enact physician antitrust exemption bills. While some critics felt unionization would encourage doctors to put their personal interests ahead of patient interests and, as a consequence, erode public trust, union proponents felt that physician collective negotiation would balance HMO and physician power more fairly and in so doing protect patients. In 1999 the AMA created its own collective bargaining unit, Physicians for Responsible Negotiation (PRN), but specifically excluded the right to strike as well as any other activity that would deny or limit treatment to patients.[10]

These various processes were the byproducts of the continuing increase in the numbers of insured individuals and families and the rapid increase in the cost of various procedures, which translated into a large increase in the dollars flowing into the health insurance industry. For-profit insurance companies used their growing financial resources to develop HMOs and other managed care entities. They ceased being enterprises that stood aloof from the delivery system, simply collecting premiums and paying bills. Now they were intimately involved with the creation of delivery systems, the interpretation of "medical need," approval of interventions, development of protocols, and monitoring of physician and hospital behavior. In response, the not-for-profit insurance sector (the Blues) developed its own HMO networks. Since the Blues did not have access to capital financing through issuance of stock, their response was less vigorous and slower. Indeed, over time many of them felt that they had to convert to for-profit status in order to compete in the capital markets and grow.

The failure during the 1970s of Presidents Nixon, Ford, and Carter to establish a national health insurance (NHI) program spurred the private sector's confidence that there would be few constraints on health care expenditures and thus on continued growth and profitability. After all, if NHI could not be legislated at a time when it was a high-priority agenda item and when there seemed to be a consensus in favor of enactment (albeit, considerable division about what to enact), the for-profits felt safe in their assumption that universal insurance and increased government control over health care expenditures were not a threat. Certainly in the 1980s there was little in a Reagan administration to lead them to feel otherwise. Indeed, they may well have felt that even were there a future administration with a different perspective on the appropriate public-private mix, they would be well established and such an important part of the health care infrastructure that they would survive. As they watched Medicare and Medicaid expenditures rise and new diagnostic, imaging, and treatment interventions continue to diffuse, they concluded that, in spite of the continuing rhetoric about the need to control costs, investments in medical care enterprises would yield good rates of return.

More access to care, an aging population, new medical interventions (including pharmaceuticals)—all these would inevitably have led to mounting expenditures. What magnified the problem, however, was the expansion in the number and scope of for-profit enterprises, and thus in market-driven behavior that sought to maximize profits. Inevitably, public concern about rising costs within the health sector became more vocal. The much-vaunted competitive market approach proved unable to stem the tide of large-scale rates of increase, always beyond, and often far beyond, that of general inflation. In addition to concerns expressed in Congress and state capitals over Medicare and Medicaid expenditures, employers who funded a significant proportion of the premiums for employed persons began to press for lower rates. They had always questioned the price of various production inputs such as labor, paper, steel, and glass; now they started questioning the level of health insurance premiums.

Employers asked what they were getting for their money. In general, they focused on both the price and the range of benefits of the health insurance they purchased; they were not yet ready to challenge the quality of the medical care their employees or beneficiaries received. Nevertheless, they were prepared to lift the veil and look behind the premium costs, that is, to examine medicine's organization and pricing structure. Payers felt they no longer had to accept the dictates of producers and insurers. They recognized that their interests and those of the insurers and of the medical care delivery systems diverged. From there, it was only a small step to question the definitions of "medically necessary" care and the quality of providers' performance. This new approach most probably was part of the erosion of the authority of professional expertise in many fields. It can be argued that this too was a legacy of Vietnam and of the student attitudes of the 1960s and early 1970s. Yesterday's students were a decade and more older. They had become "decision makers," but remained skeptical of authority and expertise.

The continuing rise in premiums intensified the instability in health care as, facing significant cost increases, employers reduced coverage (particularly for dependents); added or increased deductibles, co-insurance payments, and other cost-sharing devices; imposed additional employee contributions to premiums; and shifted contracts among providers while searching for the lowest premium in an effort to achieve short-term savings. Since insurance companies were more likely to be tied to particular managed care entities (indeed, often they were one and the same), such "churning" meant that subscribers faced discontinuities in care as well as more administrative complexity. As a consequence the battle between payers (both government and employers), deliverers, and insurers of care placed the *real* consumer, the patient, on the sidelines. In the traditional economic model there is a tension between the buyer and the seller, but the buyer is also the consumer. In medicine the tension between the purchaser and the seller still existed, but the purchaser—the employer—was not the consumer. That role belonged to the patient who, seemingly, was left out of the equation. There was little reason to believe that the purchaser truly represented the patient's needs and desires. The priorities that the potential patient set might or might not be those of the employer.

Furthermore, the seller was no longer the producer. The seller was the insurance company—insurance, after all, is what the employer was buying. The producer, however, was the physician, the allied health personnel, and the hospital and its infrastructure. The insurer did not represent those interests either. This departure from the traditional economic model that balances interests (not always in the most equitable manner) between parties with divergent interests, this confusion of roles, was among the forces making for what has been referred to as the "destabilization" of health care.[11]

The corporate structures that emerged were varied. Some for-profit hospitals and chains (as well as community not-for-profit hospitals) began to buy up medical practices. Since hospital revenues reflected the number of patients and patient days (including outpatient visits), hospitals wanted to "lock in" captive physicians, hoping (or requiring) that the physician would steer his or her patients to the hospital that had underwritten the physician's practice. Such arrangements raised issues concerning possible monopolistic practices and unethical behavior by involved physicians.[12] They also had the potential to foster unethical behavior, if, for example, the patient was led to believe that the physician was selecting the hospital appropriate to the needed care when, in fact, the selection was based on a contractual relationship or understanding.[13]

In addition to developing relationships with physicians who were expected to favor the particular hospital above others, individual hospitals and chains tried to develop their own HMO, managed care, and insurance programs. As so often proved to be the case in the world of diversification, merger, and acquisition, these corporations, which at best knew how to organize the efficient delivery of medical care (and sometimes not even that), found that they had little experience or expertise in building or running insurance ventures.[14] The issues involved in assessing risks and navigating risk selection were very different than those encountered in delivering care. The diversion of energy and resources into trying to deal with these new ventures had the potential to detract from the institutions' performance in the traditional field of medical care delivery.

The hospital industry was not alone in trying to alter existing institutional relationships and restructure the organization of the delivery system. The health insurance industry recognized that the expansion of HMOs and their variants posed an immediate and direct threat to the profitability of traditional insurance. Since HMOs combined delivery of care with insurance, their continuing expansion removed potential insurance customers from the market. Furthermore, HMOs had direct links to physicians, whose behavior and productivity they sought to control. Traditional insurers felt that they needed to develop similar relationships with members of the medical community, relationships that would balance the freedom that physicians sought with the limits that insurers needed if they were to increase their profits. Thus, as was the case in the hospital sector, insurers initiated programs that purchased physician practices or provided loan funds for office relocation or improvement. As physicians forged relationships with particular insurers, they found that they were subject to new constraints on their medical decision making.

The constraints imposed on practitioners were both direct and indirect. There were efforts to reduce utilization of services by specialists by requiring referrals from primary care physicians and by offering bonuses to these "gatekeepers" if they succeeded in keeping referrals down. There was increased monitoring of the number and frequency of diagnostic tests. Too often the physician was caught between patients who had learned about the "efficacy" of a new test from the media and the insurers who wanted to limit testing. An additional effort at cost containment called for a second opinion by another specialist if surgical or other complex procedures were contemplated. Useful as a second opinion might be, it was an additional source of discontent for physicians and patients. In some instances physicians were prohibited from informing patients about the full range of possible treatments and diagnostic options, including more costly modalities that the insurer preferred not be utilized. While these "gag" rules were seldom enforced in an effective manner, their presence was a disturbing symbol.[15]

These various attempts at control raised issues of quality. While each restraint and intervention could be defended as potentially beneficial because it might reduce the utilization of risky or unwarranted medical procedures, each could equally be criticized as potentially harmful because it might impinge on necessary or beneficial care. There was little doubt, however, that all these (and other) measures were a source of confusion and dissatisfaction for both patient and physician since, with justification, both (but especially the patient, who had less sway and less information) suspected that the rationale for the constraints was one of curbing expenditures rather than acting in the best interest of the patient.[16] Such questions were even more pointed when there were arrangements under which the physician received a bonus for achieving goals involving utilization curtailments.

The ever-closer links between the physician and the insurer and the insurer's (often successful) attempts to control and modify physician behavior raised the inevitable question: was the physician working on behalf of the insurance carrier or on behalf of the patient? A patient had reason to be as suspicious as a sports star who found himself being diagnosed and treated by the team physician employed by and answering to the franchise owner. It was not without interest that even Hollywood noted, in the film *John Q.*, that patients understand the ambiguous relationship between a physician and the insurance organization for whom the physician works.[17] The audience's knowing reaction to scenes dramatizing such conflicts underscored how the bonds of trust between patient and physician were being strained and, often, severed.

Managed Care Becomes a Force

Since each of the various new arrangements designed to alter physician behavior involved "managing" how physicians practiced medicine, the term "managed care" entered the language in the early 1980s and came to be used as an umbrella term for the many corporate arrangements under which physicians worked.[18] The tension generated by the patient's perception of the potential conflict between the physician and the insurance entity manifested itself in malpractice litigation. Patients attempted to sue corporate entities that they viewed as their health care provider only to find that though these entities set the rules, they were not the "provider" and under most circumstances could not be sued.[19] Thus patients faced a situation in which the HMO could not be held liable or accountable for the actions that it took in restricting the physician's clinical freedom.

Every aspect of the "culture" of medicine was affected by the many shifts in the relationships between patients and physicians, in the not-for-profit and for-profit character of the medical sector, and in the importance of economic considerations in structuring behavior. In less than two decades, both physicians and patients learned a new language, adopted new patterns of organization, and adapted (succumbed) to new constraints and incentives. Perhaps all this could have been anticipated. What could not have been anticipated is the remarkable speed with which, abetted with investment dollars, the delivery system with which all Americans intersected itself changed. Nor, as we have indicated, could anyone have imagined how little opposition would initially be voiced by physicians, other health professionals, and patients, even in the face of a general unhappiness. It took time for experience with these various new structures to lead to a questioning of economic theory and of the American ideology that market solutions would prove beneficent. By then the revolution, no longer an experiment, had occurred.

Federal legislation made possible the expansion of HMOs, but it was not sufficient to assure it. Though federal loan funds were made available, they involved the assumption of a debt burden. Not-for-profits had to tread cautiously, and that left ample room for the for-profit sector, which recognized the opportunity for equity investment to enter the market. In 1985, at what might (in a rough sense) be considered as the beginning of the entrepreneurial revolution, three-fourths of persons enrolled in managed care were in not-for-profit plans. By 1999 two-thirds of those enrolled were in for-profits. The founders of the prepaid group practice movement would have regarded the idea of a "for-profit" prepaid group practice as an oxymoron, but yesterday's oxymoron had become today's conventional wisdom.

The success of HMOs in the health care marketplace proved that private capital could obtain a high return. The growth in the number of HMOs and in the number of subscribers can be attributed to many factors (such as perceived quality of care, a desire for "one-stop" medicine, and consumer awareness), but the largest single factor undoubtedly was the HMO's appeal to employers and large purchasers of insurance, an appeal based on the HMO rationale and presumed economic performance, that is, on its ability to contain medical care costs and premiums. The HMO option appeared to be rational and economically logical and offered the hope of cost containment to the business community, which felt burdened by large and inexorable increases in premiums. Some analysts did argue that HMO savings were one-time gains that in greatest measure derived from a decline in hospital days per 1,000 patients. These savings did lower expenditures, but since "fat" that is trimmed once cannot be trimmed a second time, these gains could not be repeated in successive time periods. Presumably, therefore, premiums would resume their upward movement (although from a lower base). Nevertheless, cost increases appeared to ease. Much of the easing could be attributed to the lower utilization of expensive hospital days. Some of the relative stability was associated with a decline in the overall rate of inflation, and some was the result of HMO (temporary) "underpricing" policies designed to improve market share. Still, whatever the explanation, in the short run employers and employees benefited from the stabilization of premiums. Between 1991 and 1998 the annual rate of increase in health expenditures slowed to a low of 5 percent. Regrettably, it started to rise again in 1998, reaching 9.3 percent in 2002.[20] Basing the Consumer Price Index (CPI) at 100 for average prices in 1982–1984, the CPI for all nonmedical care items was 128.8 in 1990, while the CPI for medical care was 162.8, or 26.4 percent higher. By 1999 the CPI for nonmedical care items stood at 162.0, while that for medical care was 250.6, or 54.7 percent higher. The disparity continued to grow, and by 2002 the CPI for nonmedical items was 174.3, while medical care was 285.6, or 63.9 percent higher.[21]

It did prove less expensive to enroll one's employees in an HMO rather than in a traditional insurance program that offered truly "free choice." It could be even more advantageous to offer employees "premium support" at the level of the least expensive available insurance plan. In the latter case the employee paid the difference between the amount provided by the employer (most often linked to the least costly HMO) and the premium of the insurance plan the employee selected. This arrangement provided an incentive for employees to shift from fee-for-service to managed care and from a more expensive HMO to the least expensive one. Needless to say, the arrangement left many employees unhappy since they felt they were penalized if they wanted to maintain a long-standing relationship with a particular physician. Nevertheless, it should be clear that in many cases the HMO also saved money for employees. Oftentimes, it reduced (if not eliminated) cost-sharing in the form of deductibles and co-insurance. Additionally, as health costs moderated, workers were in a stronger position to press for larger wage increases.

As employers learned that they could bargain about premiums and did not have to accept the premium as set by the insurer or HMO, they tried to exert their market pressures. Negotiation over per diems and fees involved hospitals/physicians and insurers, but all parties understood that in a real sense their decisions would have to be "ratified" by employers who were paying the bill. The HMO "needed" the hospital's beds; the hospital "needed" the HMO's subscribers. Both needed the employer. The pressure to reduce premiums led to ever-stronger attempts to constrain physician and patient behavior and to limit care (more benefits initially denied, more appeals required, more patients giving up and accepting the HMO's judgments). Patient unhappiness increased when, as was often the case, the employer was offered a lower premium if he could "deliver" all employees to a single HMO and, therefore, decided to limit enrollment opportunity to that HMO and, perforce, to limit choice of physicians to those associated with that HMO.

The behaviors reflected in the dreams motivating the early founders of the prepaid group practice model could not be sustained in the face of expansion of and competition with a for-profit sector armed with very different motivations. Not-for-profits were forced to emulate the behavior and level of performance of for-profits. Nevertheless, the strongest PGPs were able to more than survive in the geographic areas in which they were already well established and accepted. The severe problems that were generated by the competitive pressures from for-profit HMOs with equity financing were most often found among the not-for-profit insurers, including the Blue Cross–Blue Shield plans, who wanted to enter the HMO market and who needed capital to do so (and even occasionally among the established PGPs when they tried to expand into new geographic areas far removed from their home base). Indeed, the pressures were such that, as noted, a number of Blue Cross–Blue Shield plans (as well as not-for-profit community hospitals) converted to for-profit status. Encouraged by state attorneys general, the proceeds of these conversions or "sales" often were used to set up "health foundations" designed to serve the public interest.[22]

The HMO, hospital, and insurance company entrepreneurial ventures already described had little continuing impact on the rate of increase in medical care costs. Efforts to ration services by establishing deterrents such as co-payments or deductibles, gatekeepers for specialist services, second opinion requirements, and limiting choice of physicians proved insufficient, ineffective, and unacceptable to the population. Furthermore, physicians began to assert themselves and argue for a greater degree of clinical independence. Patients and physicians were troubled about the trade-offs between costs, quality, and access, and forced competing HMOs to respond to these concerns and pressures. Managed care became a bit less managed; the HMO had to relax some of its constraints.

The Struggles for Efficiency, Quality, and Equity

Given the large number of insurers and for-profit entities, who were operating without a societal decision on the financing and distribution of care and who were duplicating their administrative expenses and overhead, savings that might have resulted from an efficiently organized financing mechanism did not arise. Additionally and importantly, HMOs were competing on the acquisition of the latest technology.[23] Consequently, health sector expenditures continued to escalate at rates that could not be accounted for by population growth or increases in the number of aged. It was distressing that the rise in spending took place at the same time that some forty million Americans had no private or public insurance coverage and millions more had benefits so insufficient that they would not have been able to meet the financial consequences of severe major illness.

Over the decades a universal national health insurance program had been rejected, in part because of the contention that a government plan would be complex, restrict choice, and increase costs. Now even opponents of a national universal plan had to agree that the nation seemed to have the worst of both worlds: complexity, restrictions, and cost increases without the redeeming benefit of universal coverage. The result was a sense of chaos, despair, and frustration among consumers, health professionals, and public officials.

In November 1991 Harris Wofford, a Pennsylvania Democrat, won a surprising upset victory in a special election for a vacant United States Senate seat. His success (with 55 percent of the vote) was attributed to his strong support for national health insurance: 50 percent of all

Pennsylvania voters and 64 percent of Wofford voters listed national health insurance as one of "two issues [that] mattered most in deciding how you would vote for Senator." As a consequence health insurance became an important issue in the 1992 Presidential election.[24] It was amid this political context, and the growing chaos and despair acknowledged by health care consumers, that the Clinton administration took office in 1992.

The new President, having campaigned on the need to deal with the problems of health insurance and health care, charged his wife, Hillary Rodham Clinton, with the responsibility to develop a plan for universal health insurance. Individual committees were established and convened to deal with component parts of the proposal. Press reports indicated that as many as 500 people served on these committees. The resulting plan, however, was prepared with little involvement by members of Congress—including senior members who chaired the relevant congressional committees to which emerging legislation would be referred. To say that this did not enhance the political prospects for enactment of the proposed legislation would be an understatement. Nevertheless, it would be inaccurate to suggest that the reason for failure was only that Congress was "miffed." There were substantive problems as well.

In retrospect it seems clear (and to some it appeared so at the time) that members of the executive branch and their allies lacked a sense and knowledge of history. They appeared to learn little from the fate of earlier proposals for universal coverage, such as the Carter administration proposals, which (among other things) suffered from excessive complexity. As the Clinton team tried to satisfy various interest groups as well as their own biases and priorities, their recommended legislation became ever more complicated. President Clinton rejected a "single payer" approach based on social insurance principles even as he noted that such a Canadian-like or "Medicare for all" system would be less costly than his alternative. Because he wanted to avoid tax increases and to preserve a role for insurance companies, he followed the same basic mandating approaches for employers that had been presented by President Nixon and had heavily influenced President Carter.

Of course, a single payer approach calling for new taxes and an expansion of the role of government would have been vigorously opposed by many Americans. Nevertheless, in rejecting a "Medicare for all" initiative, President Clinton rejected an approach that millions of Americans were familiar with, either as Medicare beneficiaries or family members of beneficiaries. That familiarity would have increased public understanding and perhaps (over time) public support of the legislation. The President clearly was quite prepared to call for changes in the organization and structure of the health care delivery system; he was less prepared to call for massive changes in the financial arrangements and flow and patterns of funding. But the one could not proceed smoothly without the other.

Clinton ignored perhaps the most important lesson from recent history: almost a decade elapsed between the proposal of legislation to provide health insurance for the aged and the enactment of Medicare in 1965, and that decade saw intense public education and fervent efforts from grassroots organizations. That continuing commitment and exertion helped garner support for a revolutionary change (albeit, only for part of the population) in the way the American health care system was financed. The need for public support and involvement and, in turn, the need for education and for time to undertake those activities were neglected during the Clinton effort even though the task of achieving universal health insurance was more difficult than that of enacting Medicare. True, Medicare could at best serve as an example, but the administration chose not to use that example. Instead, the President wanted to bring everyone into a program that remained employment-linked and, in that sense, would be familiar to all Americans.

But unlike the situation in pre-Medicare days when the majority of those who would be covered by Medicare were uninsured, by the 1990s most Americans already had health insurance. Furthermore, unlike Medicare, which simply provided a recognizable form of insurance plan, the Clinton proposal was designed to reorganize and change the existing delivery system. It was understandable that many Americans were troubled about a new complex proposal that they were told would be more comprehensive than what they already had, but that they had difficulty understanding. Nor had the proponents taken the formidable political expertise and resources of the health insurance industry into account. This relatively new multibillion-dollar for-profit industry used its resources to launch an extremely effective public relations campaign to defeat any legislative proposal.

The time was right for the opposition. The country had been through a long period in which successive administrations had purveyed an antigovernment ideology: that government is inefficient and wasteful, that less government is better, and that government cannot do anything right (except, perhaps, in the national security arena). The television advertising campaign by the insurance industry ("middle-Americans" Harry and Louise discussing and being puzzled by the administration's health insurance program and concluding that "there must be a better way") played upon the public distrust of government and stressed the complexity of the Clinton proposal.[25] The program details and the advertising campaign succeeded in confusing the public and in convincing a majority (both in Congress and outside the Beltway) that the plan would be both unmanageable and intrusive. Thus it was relatively easy for opponents to mount a campaign, not to amend or improve the proposed legislation, but to reject it completely. Without the grassroots education and involvement and absent congressional investment in program design, that rejection shelved the issue. The defeat of the President's initiative was thorough and complete; the matter did not come to a vote on the floor of either chamber of Congress.[26]

The large losses that the Democratic Party suffered in the congressional election of 1994 were, at least in part, attributed by political observers to the failed effort at health care reform; the public had lost faith in the Clinton administration's ability to govern and deal effectively with complex problems. Significantly, the 1994 "Contract with America," on which Republicans ran so successfully, did not include any fundamental health care reform proposals. This was the case even though the public had favored the Clinton effort when it was first proposed.[27]

Unlike Medicare legislation, which was initially defeated, but was reintroduced in session after session and thus remained on the public agenda and continued to be debated, the Clinton proposal disappeared from view. It was a one-time attempt and did not serve as a foundation for further effort. Moreover, it was a major opportunity lost and a prominent setback since the political conclusion was that national health insurance could not garner sufficient support: it was too complicated, too divisive, and those opposed could unite in opposition while those in favor split over different "favorite" priorities. The defeat of a proposal by a President who had staked so much of his and his wife's political capital on victory led many in Congress to abandon thoughts of comprehensive change and to shift their support to incremental measures. This experience, along with the brief period of decline in the rate of health expenditures in the mid-nineties, helps explain why policy makers chose to avoid developing or supporting attempts at systematic solutions for the remainder of the decade. What the distinguished social critic Elinor Langer wrote in 1967 still seemed to apply:

> I think the policy-makers are burdened by what they perceive as the enormous intellectual complexity of the task. Medical ideologists, as well as medical idealists, seem to have passed out of currency in this country, and the men now making decisions are, if anything, too modest and too humble. They number among themselves—and they certainly have access to—the best informed authorities on medical services in America and abroad. They have a clear perception of what the problems are. But they say they don't know what the answers are, or how the problems can be solved, or what they ought to do next. They are afraid of imposing overall or systematic solutions, partly because they are afraid their solutions might be wrong ones, partly because they begin with a bias against systematic solutions in general. Instead they try to do a little bit of everything at once.[28]

Nevertheless, universal health insurance is an issue that does not disappear from the public policy agenda. Though some might argue that it is an issue whose time has passed, it continues to exhibit remarkable staying power. The recent escalation in the number of Americans who lack any insurance or who have inadequate protection, combined with the continuing increase in the premiums for health insurance, is redirecting attention to the need for basic changes.[29]

The defeat of the proposed comprehensive health plan in 1993 challenged the private sector to demonstrate how well it could achieve four goals: contain costs, improve consumer satisfaction with services, provide insurance to underserved and/or uninsured populations, and increase access to care. Moreover, this challenge applied as well to publicly funded programs. While the dollars in Medicare and Medicaid flowed from government, the medical care services were provided mainly by the private sector. Yet, although all four goals or challenges posed a test of private sector efficacy, attention focused principally on the first two. Even as the number of uninsured remained relatively large (almost forty million persons, or approximately 15 percent of the population under age sixty-five),[30] the issue of universality and its relationship to equity for the most part went unaddressed. The striking decline in the number of municipal and county hospitals and beds that were publicly supported, inconsistent support for community health centers, and obstacles in maintaining Medicaid eligibility made it difficult for the poor to receive adequate continuing services. The emergency room was hardly the place to find continuity.

Incremental Initiatives

For the remainder of the last decade of the twentieth century there appeared to be no organized effective constituency pressing for a comprehensive approach to universality in coverage. Nevertheless, there were a few successful efforts to expand health insurance coverage for particular populations or target groups. One such initiative was the Health Insurance Portability and Accountability Act (HIPAA) proposed by Senators Edward Kennedy (D.-Mass.) and Nancy Kassenbaum (R.-Kans.) and enacted by Congress in 1996. HIPAA enabled individuals who had lost their employer-provided health insurance (for example, because of layoff or change in employment or in marital and/or dependent status) to continue their enrollment at their own expense. While they could not be denied insurance coverage (for example, because of preexisting conditions), subscribers had to pay the full costs of the insurance, typically without employer assistance. As with the health benefits of the Consolidated Omnibus Budget Reconciliation

Act of 1986 (COBRA), which provided similar kinds of rights to purchase insurance at group rates for certain formerly insured individuals, HIPAA protection was costly. Furthermore, the law and its relationships with COBRA[31] are exceedingly complex: the on-line booklet explaining HIPAA eligibility, benefits, exclusions, and costs runs on for fifty-two pages, and notes that each state may have additional benefits and conditions.[32]

A second initiative, arguably of much greater significance both in terms of the number of individuals involved and the degree of assistance provided, was a state child health insurance program (SCHIP), which was created by the Balanced Budget Act of 1997 under Title XXI of the Social Security Act. This measure encouraged and enabled states to initiate and to expand health insurance coverage for uninsured children. The funds covered not only the cost of insurance but also outreach services to eligible families and reasonable outlays for administration. At the end of fiscal year 2003, a total of 5.84 million children had been enrolled in SCHIP.[33] The significance of SCHIP is further illustrated by the fact that in fiscal year 2001, when some 22.7 million children were covered by Medicaid, an additional 4.6 million (20 percent) were enrolled in SCHIP. Nevertheless, SCHIP does not reach all uninsured children: as of 2001, 11 percent of all American children still had no health insurance coverage.

Still other initiatives also focused largely on mandating and improving services for the underinsured. The Women's Health and Cancer Rights Act, the Mental Health Parity Act, and the Newborns' and Mothers' Health Protection Act were all introduced and passed during this period.[34] These efforts notwithstanding, much of the attention of health policy analysts and their legislative counterparts was focused on issues of cost and quality.

The effort to deal with quality of care (and with costs) helped spawn the expansion of the field of health services research. This expansion was so rapid that it virtually created a new discipline with its own new national organization (now named AcademyHealth).[35] To a considerable extent the growth in health services research was stimulated by the increasing application of epidemiological and biostatistical methods in biomedical research. The creative studies by Professor Archie

Cochrane[36] had furthered the method of randomized clinical trials. In time such trials in which patients were assigned to different treatment modalities became the "gold standard" for evaluating the effectiveness of new diagnostic and therapeutic interventions and were important in attracting the funds and personnel necessary to advance the field. In addition to randomized clinical trials, epidemiologic studies galvanized both understanding and practice. Using the tools of epidemiology the report of the Surgeon-General's Advisory Committee on Smoking and Health in 1964 had established the causation of lung cancer by cigarette smoking and provided new information and hope to millions of individuals.[37] Now these approaches led to attempts to see "what works" and at what cost and to "evidence-based medicine." Practitioners and patients were becoming much more knowledgeable and sophisticated on matters of health care.

Understandably a large influx of professionals (physicians, public health experts, economists, epidemiologists, statisticians, political scientists, lawyers, and MBAs, among others) was drawn into research on effectiveness, efficacy, and quality. The universities, especially the schools of public health, institutionalized the field in departments of health services research and/or management. In the private sector there was an increase in the number of consulting groups ready, willing, and (claiming to be) able to provide data and studies to evaluate various components of medical care as well as to advise payers and third-party reimbursers for medical care.

Much of the research and evaluation in health services focused on effectiveness, efficiency, and quality. In considerable measure these studies hoped to provide a basis for reducing utilization of "unnecessary" or cost-ineffective health care services and, as a result, moderating the rate of increase in health expenditures. On the face of it one might wonder why individual institutions or individual physicians would welcome such research: after all, moderation in expenditures would mean that the pie to be shared by providers would be smaller than would otherwise be the case. Such considerations were outweighed by a number of possible factors: a feeling that continued rapid expansion in health expenditures would lead to government intervention and price controls; a conviction that health care was not a zero-sum game, that there would be continued expansion of efficacious interventions as a consequence of biomedical research; a continued belief in a medical "ethic" and "ethos"; and a view that in a competitive world institutions could gain at the expense of others by demonstrating their commitment to effectiveness and efficiency and thus make up for the decline in the size of the pie by getting a much larger slice, that is, market share.

"Effectiveness and efficiency" related directly to the quality of medical care, to the ability to provide more and better care with existing resources. The increased emphasis on quality, in part the result of pressures brought by more knowledgeable consumers (read: patients) who were less willing to accept "authority," led to a growing body of research on medical errors. The Institute of Medicine of the National Academy of Science published two reports: *To Err Is Human* in 1999[38] and *Crossing the Quality Chasm* in 2001.[39] Both attracted wide attention and provided evidence that for the most part "errors" were not the failure of individual providers, but of systems.[40] While systems are hard to alter, the benefits of change can be far-reaching. New data systems, computers, and an increased willingness to rely on electronic assists in such areas as medical record keeping and ordering and filling of pharmaceutical prescriptions seemed to offer hope for a reduction in the large number of deaths and injuries associated with error.[41]

Interest intensified in these and related issues, including the pioneering studies by John Wennberg and his associates on the wide geographic variation in patterns of practice, variations that could not be defended on scientific grounds. The level of interest was such that it inspired the establishment, within the Department of Health and Human Services, of the Agency for Healthcare Research and Quality (AHRQ),[42] which conducts its own studies, provides funding for extramural investigations, and serves as a focal point for these various concerns within government. Medicine's scientific base was now spreading beyond the learned journals and the halls of the medical school into the delivery of health care services.

Even as there was an increased emphasis on system effectiveness and efficiency, there also was increased attention to interventions designed to alter patient behavior. This interest had begun as early as the mid-1970s during a period of rapid growth in health care prices and health care expenditures. Advances in computer technology and the implementation of ever more sophisticated statistical techniques enabled an expansion of rigorous research into the impact of risk factors and "lifestyle" on health. In turn, however (in keeping with the economic adage that for every benefit there is a cost, though, we hasten to add, not necessarily a commensurate one), these new investigations and the implications of their findings raised issues of privacy and the confidentiality of patient information.

There is no gainsaying that the emphasis on lifestyle changes and prevention (around such issues as smoking, exercise, and nutrition) was beneficial, even if, on occasion, it was stimulated by an attempt to reduce utilization, medical care expenditures, and public and collective responsibility and action. These interventions to modify health behavior were strengthened in the 1990s and were accompanied by various efforts, some of them quite appropriate, directed at discouraging patients from utilizing services unnecessarily. Often these programs aimed at changing high-risk behaviors did not require physician input. Thus patients (especially those who were enrolled in HMOs modeled after the original PGPs) became more familiar with triage and encounters with professionals without an "M.D." after their name.

The emphasis on controlling costs led to other interventions, some with more problematic outcomes. Thus, for example, many insurance programs introduced or increased the levels of co-payments, co-insurance, and deductibles associated with each rendered service. These programs were designed to increase patient cost-consciousness, but had the obvious additional advantage (for the employer, who most often was the payer) of reducing employer premium expenditure. If utilization did not change, the advantage would not be a reduction in total costs, but, with funds coming out of multiple "pockets," a reduction in perceived outlays. When utilization did decline, that raised the question whether such programs not only discouraged "unnecessary visits," but also visits that provided desirable preventive and early diagnosis services.[43] Always there was the nagging equity issue: the impact of cost-sharing initiatives hit unevenly as a consequence of the significant income disparities found in the insured population. The modest number of out-of-pocket dollars required for cost-sharing might provide a meaningless disincentive for the CEO, but a meaningful disincentive for his or her secretary.

Still other efforts to control costs were directed at insurance program characteristics and, it was hoped, through them at subscriber behavior. Thus, since HMOs continued to be viewed as "efficient" mechanisms to reduce expenditures (or at least to moderate increases), there was an attempt to induce Medicare beneficiaries to shift from Medicare fee-for-service to HMOs. Under this "Medicare + Choice" program, the government would pay a capitated amount (somewhat larger than the average Medicare per beneficiary cost) to the HMO, and the HMO would provide all the Medicare benefits to the enrollee and, in addition, other benefits (for example, drug coverage) that would appeal to subscribers. HMOs were attracted to this venture and all the more so since, in spite of regulations requiring "open" enrollment, they were able (through adroit "cream skimming" and "cherry picking") to add healthier subscribers. Their advertisements stressed fitness and well-being and often had photographs of elders playing golf, swimming, and otherwise participating in physical exercise programs. Conversely, there were reasons to believe that few encouragements were offered to disabled and other individuals with above-average needs or risks.

Of course, beneficiaries who were disabled, frailer, older, and sicker and who had long-standing relationships with their physicians were less likely to change doctors and enroll in the HMO. As a consequence, with the healthiest patients siphoned out of the general risk pool, the average costs in the traditional Medicare fee-for-service program rose. In turn, because of "linkage," the law, as written, called for higher payments to the HMOs. The Medicare program realized that because premiums were not adjusted to take account of risk selection, instead of saving money by expanding HMO enrollment, Medicare was actually spending more. Yet, even as Medicare felt that it was paying excessive amounts to the HMOs, a growing number of HMOs felt that they were receiving insufficient payments and dropped out of the program. From 1999 to 2003, HMOs dropped 2.4 million Medicare beneficiaries (mostly from Medicare + Choice plans). As of September 2003, 4.6 million Medicare beneficiaries were enrolled in HMOs, down from a peak of 6.3 million in 1999.[44] Karen Ignagni, president of the American Association of Health Plans, claimed that with health care inflation growing at 12 percent and Medicare reimbursement increases capped at 2 percent, few HMOs could afford to continue participating in Medicare.[45]

What had been an initiative to reduce Medicare expenditures (and improve beneficiary benefits out of the "extra" rewards the HMOs were receiving) did not turn out to be the answer to Medicare's budget problems. The implication of this attempt reverberated and became a fractious issue in the 2003 debates around Medicare reform. The "reform" ultimately adopted once again emphasizes "choice" (now renamed "Medicare Advantage") and provides significantly higher subsidies to managed care organizations in an effort to entice them back into the program.

The reader may be confused by this development. If HMOs are better or more efficient, why is it necessary to provide a handsome subsidy to induce them to enroll subscribers? How does paying the HMO more than the average Medicare beneficiary costs (perhaps significantly more, after the subsidy and the relative risk of the enrolled population are taken into account) save money for the Medicare system? It is quite reasonable to find this kind of economic reasoning confusing. The explanation lies in the fact that in adopting Medicare Advantage ideology trumped economics.

The law is written so that all programs, including traditional Medicare, have to compete. As time passes and individuals change their enrollment to reflect their health risks, and thus remove themselves from the larger community group, two things occur: (1) the "social fabric" on which Medicare relies is torn asunder as individuals view themselves as "belonging" to an HMO and not to Medicare; (2) with favorable risk selection, HMOs that enroll Medicare beneficiaries flourish, and as they grow and premiums in traditional Medicare rise and enrollment declines it becomes much easier to evolve to a voucher system, even one that is income-related. That, of course, would end social insurance Medicare as we know it. Dr. Fein remembers well a day-long health economics seminar two colleagues and he held for some half-dozen senior White House and Executive Office staff members of the Nixon administration. With only one exception they considered Medicare to be "bad policy" and a mistake. In their view helping the aged poor was appropriate (they truly were "compassionate conservatives"), but enacting a universal social insurance program that covered all the aged was not. Now, over three decades later, their views were embodied in legislation that negates the value of social cohesion and could lead to a less universal and very different kind of Medicare program.

It is clear that the costs of the Medicare program will increase as a consequence of Medicare Advantage (certainly at least in the short run). Proponents and opponents were divided over issues of competition, privatization, and the long-run implications for the traditional Medicare program that many beneficiaries prefer. Given the cost implications, it is undoubtedly fair to conclude that those who favor the Medicare changes that were adopted do so because of a deep-seated belief about the virtues of private competition. That HMOs require a large subsidy to compete effectively with the fee-for-service sector and that this subsidy will have significant (unfavorable) budget implications are ignored. So, too, the fact that this dependence on subsidy is at odds with the kind of "level playing field" associated with effective competition.

Earlier we referred to the efforts to contain costs by constraining what physicians could do: refusing to approve proposals for hospitalization or costly procedures, requiring second opinions, and even enforcing "gag" rules. The implementation of these various efforts required setting up complex administrative structures, which in turn added to administrative costs. Personnel and expenditures continued to increase[46] even as both patients and physicians felt more and more oppressed. The dissatisfaction became so generalized that in 1999 the large insurer, United Healthcare, abandoned various requirements and indicated it would abide by physicians' judgments.[47] Subsequently, Aetna adopted new standards designed to reduce physician hostility (and litigation) and, as an important byproduct, to benefit subscribers. But it is unclear whether these "relaxed" standards will be maintained in the face of continuing increases in costs.

In a sense these efforts represent a recognition that the health care

system operated with a confusing set of conflicting objectives: employers and government wanted to contain costs; insurers felt they had to
respond to those demands and control premiums; patients, impressed
by the explosion in medical knowledge and information, wanted the
benefits of new medical care advances; and physicians wanted to practice medicine under conditions that maximized their clinical freedom.
No single health care institution could resolve those conflicts. While
some assumed that government could and would do so, it was not evident that was possible. Government presumably represented the people, but the people offered no clear direction. Influenced by lobbyists,
ideology, and campaign funding, the nation's representatives were unable and unwilling to provide the leadership and education over a sustained period of time to force choice between competing goals and visions. Inevitably, there was a high level of frustration, except perhaps
among those (by and large the more affluent) who preferred the status
quo.

The reader undoubtedly may conclude that both private and public
health policy have been moving back and forth and subject to a good
deal of "churning." That certainly was the case. Nevertheless, despite
all the difficulties—with the distribution of health care, the share of
the GDP devoted to health expenditures, and the changing ethos of
medicine as for-profit entrepreneurs came to play a greater role—
there were significant advances in health. Could we have done even
better? Most assuredly, the answer is yes. That, however, does not negate the progress that did take place. It is to those matters that we now
turn.

6 | Beyond the Dollars:
Progress in Health and the
Role of Public Health

The public certainly has many valid reasons to value health care services. Nonetheless, as in earlier time periods, major improvements in vital statistics are due to factors that can be considered outside the medical care delivery system. Improvements in living conditions, nutrition (albeit, the latter increasingly offset by obesity), and environment, as well as changes in behavior (for example, the decline in smoking and increase in exercise) have made the actual difference. Efforts to quantify the impact of medical care have suggested that perhaps it accounts for 10 percent of the improvements to public health.[1] Given the very large economic disparities in the United States and their influence on living conditions, this should not come as a surprise.

Nevertheless, the preoccupation of both the general public and policy makers with biomedical research was understandable. Its achievements were dramatic and, in many cases, had a science-fiction-like quality as researchers created ever more potent diagnostic and therapeutic tools transforming the practice of medicine. The applications of basic knowledge led to advances in genetics and in reproductive biology; the developments in immunology increased the feasibility of organ transplantation; and exciting imaging techniques and related technologies made laparoscopic surgery possible. Interventions based on these and other innovations, undreamt of several decades ago, were institutionalized and became commonplace. Since they often involved new equipment and new pharmaceuticals, there were reasons for their producers and associated public relations departments to seek media coverage. This was forthcoming, and television, magazines, and newspapers featured the dramatic success stories, both in their news and, increasingly, in their business sections.

Despite a commitment to the continuing quest to understand disease processes and discover potential cures, biomedical research scientists were also moving toward new intellectual frontiers and investigative interests that emphasized techniques for early detection of disease and preventive medicine.[2] The quantitative methods of epidemiology and biostatistics, together with biomedical knowledge, made the development of screening methods for early diagnosis possible and led to the expectation that treatment outcomes would be improved. Some screening tests, such as for the identification of phenylketonuria (PKU) in newborn infants, proved their effectiveness in preventing mental retardation. Others, such as mammography for early detection of breast cancer, remained subject to continuing scrutiny.

Part of the debate involved the frequency of false negatives (the failure to recognize the disease when it was present) and of false positives (a test result that "found" the disease when, in fact, it was not present). Part of the debate related to whether "success" is measured by a change in life expectancy (and if so, is the measure the benefit that the relatively few "winners" gain, say five years, or the benefit averaged over all individuals, including those who do not benefit at all, thus reducing the average benefit considerably?). We were caught in the old argument: if the chances of "success" are only one in a hundred, does one reject the procedure or go forward, convinced that this individual may be the "one"? Society's perspective and that of the individual patient or physician may differ. Furthermore, as has been argued in relation to heart bypass surgery, perhaps life expectancy is an inappropriate measure. Perhaps success should be measured by improvement in the quality of life (though it is unclear how and by whom that is to be calibrated).

The growing interest of biomedical research workers in early detection of disease and in prevention, as well as the gains in the science knowledge base and in the sophistication of research methodologies, provided reasons to anticipate the opportunity for more effective interventions. These trends were predicted over thirty years ago.[3] Nevertheless, it was not evident that these opportunities would be translated into more effective medical care programs and treatments. The application of the new knowledge required both a social strategy and political will.

The expansion of knowledge, the media attention, and the increasing level of health expenditures combined to create greater public awareness not only about the world of medicine in general, but about specific diseases and possible cures. Following the extraordinary success of the March of Dimes in mobilizing the public's financial support for efforts that culminated in a polio vaccine, many similar voluntary health organizations were founded that, in addition to fund raising and education, became advocates for larger budgetary allocations to the National Institutes of Health (NIH). In the process the public became informed about health issues and learned to work with health professionals. In relation to the NIH and to the broad agenda of fighting various diseases, the general public and thousands of concerned volunteers were replicating the earlier relationship of President Franklin Delano Roosevelt to the March of Dimes and poliomyelitis. While the proliferation of these organizations resulted in some inevitable fragmentation, and though some health professionals protested that they created a "disease-of-the-month" climate, their collective efforts undoubtedly had an important impact on raising consciousness about health improvement.[4]

These efforts mirrored the pluralism of our society and therefore were not orderly. Nevertheless, it is difficult to believe that a more careful or coordinated effort would have been more influential in regard to the NIH budget or more beneficial in regard to public health education. These organizations of "outsiders" provided a voice for individuals and families who were experiencing health problems or were especially sensitive to particular health issues and, importantly, for those who were paying the taxes that supported the various federal, state, and local health initiatives. Voluntary health organizations were (and remain) an integral part of our democratic processes. While they sometimes prove to be an irritant to the "experts," their presence and active participation help fund those very experts, enabling them to pursue their work.

In the late 1990s the lobbying efforts by the public and strong congressional interest in medical research led to a commitment to double the NIH budget over a five-year period. This pledge was met, and the 2003 appropriation was $27 billion.[5] To some extent this action reflected a congressional desire to demonstrate a concern for the health of the American people while camouflaging the harsh political reality that efforts to guarantee universal access to health insurance and to curb the rise in health expenditures continued to founder. Funding research was ideologically acceptable to members of both parties: the days when federal research subsidies were viewed negatively as government intrusion had long since passed. Finally, though large, NIH appropriations were less than 2 percent of total health expenditures and about 5 percent of federal health expenditures. Conversely, dealing with expenditure control, health care delivery, insurance, and planning and rationalization issues would have been far more costly and divisive. These involved differing views on federalism, the relative size and scope of government and of the private health sector, and the role of social insurance.

It should, of course, be acknowledged that for many members of legislatures, as well as for the public, support for research had merit in and of itself. It offered the hope of successful intervention in pressing and often distressing health conditions, many of which had personally touched those very legislators. Furthermore, as previously noted, appropriations to NIH spoke to a deep-seated belief that the answer to all problems lay in technology and American know-how. Although a growing interest by medical research workers in prevention and early detection of disease moved the field closer to a population-based public health perspective, by and large the medical profession, as well as medical education, remained focused on the improvement of clinical care.[6]

The reports of scientific advances were exciting and most welcome, even if the reports often noted that it might take years to fully document the findings, develop the clinical applications, conduct the necessary clinical trials, and move the science from the laboratory into practice at the patient's bedside—the latter step qualified by the proviso that the new therapy turn out to be "affordable." Yet, somewhat under the radar and certainly with fewer headlines, vital statistics were showing quite remarkable improvement. These changes were part of the "quiet triumph of public health," a triumph that took place even as the public health sector was underfunded and as the public health infrastructure was being weakened. Federal, state, and local government expenditures for all public health activities (including health promotion and disease prevention) were only about 11 percent of total health expenditures.

Ambiguities in the Shaping of Health Policy

Among the crucial contributions to the health of the population were those made under the aegis of the Office of the Surgeon-General, which served as the focal point for federal endeavors in public health campaigns and education. The first national action campaign, led by Dr. Thomas Parran in the 1930s, was designed to control venereal disease.[7] The 1964 report of the Surgeon-General's Advisory Committee on Smoking and Health to Dr. Luther Terry has had an enduring impact. In 1979 *Healthy People: The Surgeon-General's Report on Health Promotion and Disease Prevention* (often referred to simply as *Healthy People*), established decennial quantitative health goals for the nation and provided a framework for action across the spectrum of health issues.

The role of the Surgeon-General and the influence of his or her office on public health education and practice became more visible and significant in the 1980s with the unexpected emergence of the AIDS epidemic.[8] Not only does the Surgeon-General have the opportunity to set the public agenda on health matters (though, perhaps, not in such areas as the organization and financing of health care), he or she also participates in the coordination of the public health activities of the various agencies in the United States Public Health Service, the NIH, the Centers for Disease Control, the Food and Drug Administration, the Alcohol, Drug Abuse, and Mental Health Administration, and the Health Resources and Services Administration, each of which has educational and/or regulatory responsibilities. It is appropriate to note that over the decade of the nineties the Secretary of the Department of Health and Human Services (HHS) came to play an increasingly significant role as a spokesperson for public health and particularly so after 1995 when the Social Security Administration (SSA) became an independent agency.

While HHS and its constituent agencies were most visible in dealing with health policy and programs, similar activity was found in other departments. This was both an asset and a problem; it provided broader auspices to improve health, but also diffused responsibility.

Regulatory agencies such as the Environmental Protection Agency, the Federal Trade Commission, the Federal Aviation Administration, and the National Transportation Safety Board all had significant responsibilities in the health field, as did the Departments of Veterans Affairs (administering numerous health benefit and service programs), Defense (addressing service personnel and their dependents), Agriculture (especially in relation to food and nutrition issues), Labor (focusing, through the Occupational Safety and Health Administration, on workers' health), and the Treasury (especially in relation to matters involving the tax code and its relationship to medical deductions and premium support), as well as, among others, the Departments of Transportation, Energy, and State.

In addition, much health policy is developed and implemented in the private sector. We have already addressed the role of the insurance industry as a major force in generating measures that influence the lives of many people. In addition, in keeping with the American pluralistic tradition, many nongovernmental health organizations and community-based health organizations play significant roles in shaping the national health agenda. Indeed, as we have pointed out, the continuing growth of the NIH over the decades can be attributed in part to well-organized support from the private sector, which had a major impact on generating public as well as congressional favor for biomedical research.[9] Thus policies developed in the health arena are an inevitable collaboration between the public and private sectors. This is not unexpected since our delivery system is largely private, though the financing for much of its activity (for example, through Medicare and Medicaid) is largely public.

In their report, *Health Policies for the 21st Century: Challenges and Recommendations for the U.S. Department of Health and Human Services,* Jo

Ivey Boufford and Phillip Lee explain how health policies result from multiple sources diffused among public and private organizations and agencies. They state:

Divided responsibilities in Washington create and reinforce overlapping and competing jurisdictions in state and local governments and among myriad private-sector stakeholders. Federal health-related agencies lack effective working relationships that cross organizational boundaries and make possible effective coordination of either the work of federal, state, and local agencies or collaboration of public agencies with the corporate sector and community-based organizations.

Within the DHHS there is inadequate coordination of the agencies of the Public Health Service (PHS). The department also needs more knowledge of the challenges facing its stakeholders, especially non-governmental organizations, advocacy groups, grantees, and business groups as they work to promote health.[10]

In spite of the diffuseness of the responsibility for health policies at the federal level, the Secretary of the Department of Health and Human Services is generally regarded as the central figure for shaping priorities within the health agenda. This is not unwarranted, since the Centers for Medicare and Medicaid Services (CMS) under HHS account for more than a quarter of the total national health care expenditures and a much higher percentage of federal health expenditures.[11] Since the Secretary has responsibility for the NIH (which spends over 40 percent of the HHS discretionary budget)[12] as well as the other operating agencies of the Public Health Service (PHS), he or she is called upon to make recommendations furthering public health.

Importantly, there was an increasing recognition that the federal role in advancing health extended far beyond paying the bills for Medicare beneficiaries and providing funds to the states to do the same for Medicaid recipients. In the period after 1966, when both programs were implemented at the federal level (the implementation of state Medicaid programs depended on state initiatives and, therefore, took place at different times), government viewed itself as a bill payer. Indeed, in section 1801 ("Prohibition against any Federal interference") the original Medicare legislation virtually repeated the language of the

Ways and Means Committee report in stating that "nothing in this title shall be construed to authorize any Federal officer or employee to exercise any supervision or control over the practice of medicine or the manner in which medical services are provided, or over the selection, tenure, or compensation of any officer or employee of any institution, agency, or person providing health services; or to exercise any supervision or control over the administration or operation of any such institution, agency, or person."[13]

As time passed, it became clear that the massive expenditures under both Medicare and Medicaid could not be "neutral," that, inevitably, they would affect medical practice and, further, that government had a responsibility, to patients and taxpayers alike, to make certain that it was receiving "value for money." Thus, in a newer configuration, the Health Care Financing Administration (HCFA) began to examine efficacy and quality and to behave as if it was purchasing care, not merely paying bills. CMS (which replaced HCFA) has continued to operate under that philosophy. Indeed, most insurers in the private sector have adopted that paradigm as well.

Augmenting the variety of public programs at the federal level were programs at the state and local level. In general, health goals set by the federal government were taken seriously and given a high priority by state and local health departments even though many of them were experiencing chronic and serious budgetary problems. Because many of the various local and state efforts were more attuned to the challenges of chronic care as contrasted with acute care and lacked the sense of drama associated with epidemics and pandemics, it was difficult for them to receive adequate funding.

As health policy issues became more complex and rose higher on the national agenda, a consensus developed among health professionals that a national institution was needed to conduct studies to help policy makers. The logical setting for such an enterprise seemed to be the National Academy of Sciences, which had been chartered by Congress during the Civil War to assist governmental agencies in formulating science policy. In 1967 the Board of the National Academy of Sciences responded by appointing a Board on Medicine, which was redesignated the Institute of Medicine (IOM) in 1970. From its creation it has been committed to a number of objectives, importantly including the development of "knowledge and policies that improve health for present and future generations."[14]

Perhaps the IOM's most important contributions are the studies and reports it generates to inform policy makers. Because its membership is geographically and professionally diverse, these reports add up to an eclectic approach to the analysis of policy issues. Due to the IOM's charter, the reports are not advocacy documents, but instead are intended to produce balanced analyses. An overview of the reports provides a useful guide to the health policy issues facing the nation.

As early as 1988 the Institute of Medicine expressed its concern about the failure to maintain the level of investment required to support the public health infrastructure and warned that it was weakening.[15] The gradual erosion of the public health systems assumed greater significance as a consequence of the attacks on the World Trade Center on September 11, 2001. Worries about possible bioterrorism attacks, while emphasizing potential threats by specific infectious agents and toxins,[16] highlighted the importance of rebuilding basic public health structures, capacities, and competencies. Since the nature of a potential bioterrorist attack is not predictable, a generic competence of the public health system is needed in order to offer the best protection.

The problem of adequate support for public health is representative of a more general problem involving the allocation of resources and the balancing of long-run and short-run goals and strategies. During a period of crisis an emphasis on acquiring answers to perceived but unknown threats may distort the setting of priorities. Thus earmarking funds specifically for important research on bioterrorism (out of a fixed public health budget) runs the risk of diverting efforts away from major long-term public health threats such as AIDS, malaria, tuberculosis, and the diarrheal diseases. Maintaining publicly funded research on these diseases is important, since these are not priority matters for the pharmaceutical industry because the populations at risk and many of the countries in which they reside are predominantly poor and the development of new drugs would not yield a high rate of return. Clearly, what is required is an increase in the total public health budget, not a shifting around of inadequate funds.

The concerns involving population health required the perspectives that had guided public health activities and the specific application, developed over many decades, of disciplines and methodologies such as epidemiology. Medical schools and their associated hospitals and outpatient services necessarily focused on teaching students in the context of caring for the individual patient—population health was not central to their mission. Conversely, schools of public health, free of the responsibility for large-scale clinical services and resources, could focus more on health promotion and disease prevention. Their locus of activity was the community, not the bedside. The various reports by the Surgeons-General, the Institute of Medicine, and others were appearing and becoming influential just as the first revolution in public health (the decline of the acute infectious diseases) was coming to an end. It therefore is useful to examine the unique role the schools of public health played in this epidemiologic transition.

In contrast to medical schools, which had achieved a high degree of educational standardization in order to assure the clinical competence of all physicians, from their inception schools of public health retained their heterogeneity with a range of models and goals. While the Association of Schools of Public Health had established an accreditation process, its objective was to assure the quality of instruction and not the standardization of the curriculum. Nevertheless, there was considerable agreement that certain curricular contents were important for the development of greater research competence and for training health workers to lead and manage public health and medical care programs in the public and private sectors.

While departmental structures varied, all schools emphasized quantitative skills, the health of populations, management and finance, and international health issues.[17] In addition, schools understood the need to have students with diverse educational and occupational backgrounds. Consequently, physicians, nurses, dentists, pharmacists, and other health professionals were enrolled in course work with economists, political scientists, sociologists, anthropologists, social workers, and other social scientists, as well as with students from engineering, law, and other disciplines who were finding outlets for their interests in the expanding health sector. Furthermore, enrollment of students from different countries at different stages of economic development, with different health systems, levels of resources, culture, traditions, and health problems, enriched the educational experience of all students even as it reflected the fact that, with increased mobility, disease patterns could and did spread rapidly across national boundaries.

Biomedical Sciences, Academic Health Centers, and the Spawning of the Medical Industrial Complex

The scientific revolution that was set in motion shortly following World War II resulted in continued growth in the biomedical sciences throughout the rest of the century.[18] While few research efforts were as dramatic as the discovery of the double-helix arrangement of DNA for a basic understanding of genetics (for which the Nobel Prize was awarded to James Watson, Francis Crick, and Maurice Wilkins in 1954), there was considerable research creativity in the basic sciences.

It was fortunate that the leadership of the National Institutes of Health emphasized research in the basic sciences even when there were great pressures for more focus on applied research. NIH took seriously the admonition of Dr. Alvin Weinberg, director of the Oak Ridge National Laboratory, who, in responding to a challenge by President Johnson in 1966, asserted that since the bulk of biomedical research was in the prefeasibility stage, the underlying basic research had to be broad. He argued that the vital link between basic and applied biomedical research was much more haphazard and unpredictable than he suspected the President would have wished, and went on to state that most basic molecular biologists would rather work directly on a cure for cancer than on whatever they were then doing, and would have done so if only they knew how to make real progress.[19] Though this view about the importance of basic science and research prevailed, it inevitably made for difficulties in dealing with Presidents and legislators who wanted to be able to tell taxpayers about dramatic successes in applied areas.

The basic sciences flourished under expanded NIH funding, providing the fundamental knowledge that, in turn, allowed applied research and development to thrive. And indeed, even though (because of the number of persons affected) the beneficial results may not be apparent in examining the vital statistics, they are very apparent to many individuals and families: some cancers and other illnesses are now curable; the quality of life has been improved for many persons. Furthermore, advances in the basic sciences and in our understanding of genetics and of disease processes point to even greater future possibilities.

In addition to generating national support for the growth of the biomedical research enterprise, the NIH planners allocated funds for research training. This both created pressure for and made possible the continued expansion of research. While the training was initially predominantly targeted for physicians to enable them to become clinical investigators, over time the numbers of trainees from other fields multiplied. In recent years, particularly as medical training has become lengthier and costlier, there is concern about a decline in the number of physicians electing to enter research training and, thus, a potential decline in clinical investigation.[20]

The creativity of this research and all its applications are far too numerous and beyond the scope of this discussion. Nevertheless, several important and exciting categories are worth noting: (1) the advances in genetics and the mapping of the entire human genome; (2) the much greater understanding of immunology; (3) gains within the neurosciences; (4) improvements in technology; (5) possibilities involving stem-cell research; and (6) achievements in epidemiology and biostatistics. Also of relevance is the evolving utilization of the Internet for communication, research, and interaction with patients.[21] The impressive progress within the biomedical sciences had a remarkable impact on the health science centers of the academic community. Just as NIH growth fostered an expanding research effort within universities, medical schools, and hospitals (and more recently within HMOs and other ambulatory health delivery systems), so the expansion of research in health-related industries also spilled back into the academic world. Instruments, devices, pharmaceuticals, and telecommunication technologies needed development and evaluation, and faculty members were increasingly being asked to participate in such industry-supported applied research.

Understandably, perhaps inevitably, conflicts of interests developed.

As long as research support came from NIH, faculty members needed to compete for grants, but had no financial conflicts of interest. That an investigator might report success simply in order to increase the likelihood of a second or third grant was certainly possible; while not numerous, examples of such research fraud did surface. An important although not perfect protection against such dishonesty was the publication of results in peer-reviewed journals so that colleagues could replicate experiments. By definition, there were no "trade secrets," and findings were shared with colleagues and, most appropriately, with students. The research world of the university and of the medical school was based on openness and trust. In part, the competitive but generally collegial atmosphere that prevailed undoubtedly reflected the fact that health care had not yet emerged as a major sector of the economy. The university was smaller, research activities were at a different (and lesser) scale, there were not so many dollars and, it may be said, fewer temptations. Those were the days when faculty members spoke of "psychic income."

However, when the research enterprise and the number of dollars in the health care system "exploded" and industry support suddenly materialized, many potential and real conflicts arose. First, a number of faculty members saw the possible profitability of the many new devices and drugs under development, and sought and acquired patents. They could commercialize these by direct sale to industry, through royalties, and/or through stock options. In addition, with the help of venture capital, some academics established new firms, contributing to the growth and development of the biotechnology industry. Since research findings had important financial repercussions on the particular firms that had sponsored the research, work that had previously been shared with students and colleagues often came to be viewed as falling under the rubric of trade secrets. The entrepreneur-investigator was placed (and placed him- or herself) in a curious competing role of being a university "employee" and yet having a financial interest in behaving as an employee of the sponsoring commercial establishment. This was a very far cry from the days in 1925 when Professor Henry Steenbock of the University of Wisconsin (Madison) helped stimulate the development of the University of Wisconsin Alumni Research

Foundation (WARF). This organization was designed to manage patents on UW-Madison inventions in a manner that would assure that they would be used for public benefit and bring any financial gains back to the university for further research. Professor Steenbock turned over his patent in the field of Vitamin D (to combat rickets) to WARF. Since 1928, when it made its first grant, WARF has given $750 million to fund research.[22]

The concern over conflicts of interest became sufficiently widespread that medical editors began to write editorials about the medical-industrial complex. In September 2001, eleven major medical journals agreed to require disclosures of financial interests of authors, and established codes under which authors were required to declare the source of funding for their work.[23] Even so, these problems of peer review became more difficult since many "peers" themselves had commercial connections.[24] In medical schools, and more generally in universities, efforts were made to codify acceptable standards of conduct concerning for-profit support and activities by faculty members.[25]

The growing commercialization of the biomedical enterprise was particularly evident in the pharmaceutical industry's use of swelling advertising budgets to expand its sales.[26] In 1997 the industry persuaded the Food and Drug Administration (FDA) to relax its rules governing the promotion of prescription drugs to the public.[27] Despite industry claims that such advertising was informational and designed to create "educated consumers," it does not stretch credulity to suggest its true purpose was to increase the probability that patients would press their physicians to prescribe the drugs that had been touted.

Commercialization was further evident in the reporting of medical developments in the business sections and on the financial pages of the newspapers. As hospital corporations, health insurers, and managed care companies, as well as drug and device manufacturers, grew larger and as their stock was traded on the financial markets, the details of new research developments that might influence corporate earnings regularly appeared in the financial columns. The business pages were the places to turn to to learn about the most recent hospital "strategic plan," the latest biomedical advances (or what purported to be advances), FDA approval or disapproval of pharmaceuticals and de-

vices, and the stock market prospects of varying enterprises. Capti-
vated by even the skimpiest reports of early clinical trials, subject to
the hype and spin of public relations departments, we seemed to be
developing a culture that behaved as if medicine had the answer to all
health problems and that if it didn't have those answers today, it surely
would have them tomorrow. The media fed our appetites, and contributed to increases in both health awareness and health expenditures.

The Protection of Human Subjects

Historically, the protection of human subjects in clinical studies was
based on an informal reliance on the ethical codes of individual professional conduct as well as the standards of professional organizations
and institutional safeguards. Over time there was ample evidence that
this informal system was very far from perfect (indeed, far from adher-
ing to any reasonably acceptable standard). The public, learning about
earlier gross violations of ethical standards, recognized the unmistak-
able fallibility of scientists, some of whom were apparently so enam-
ored of their endeavors that they were willing to place human beings
at considerable known or suspected risk in order to obtain more data
and richer research results. Perhaps the most prominent example was
the conduct of a study on the natural history of syphilis in which the
subjects enrolled were denied the benefit of penicillin therapy when it
became available.[28] There were similar revelations concerning studies in which individuals were exposed to radiation hazards.[29] In part
as a reaction to these "experiments," and out of awareness that the
numbers of investigators and clinical studies were rising—as was the
number of cases involving "misbehavior"—the prevailing informal arrangements came under closer scrutiny and were deemed to be inadequate.

As the largest funder of biomedical research, the NIH required that
each institution under whose auspices research proposals were submitted establish an institutional review board (IRB) to protect human
subjects. The IRB had to examine each proposal to determine that it
met appropriate ethical safeguards.[30] The boards were to be composed
of public representatives as well as health professionals and research

workers. In order to facilitate clinical trials conducted by the pharmaceutical industry, institutional review boards were also set up that were independent of and unaffiliated with any university or research institute. In general, these IRBs were managed by for-profit corporations funded by the pharmaceutical industry.

While the monitoring of the protection of human subjects and disciplinary action for ethical violations remained largely within the universities, the Department of Health and Human Services, which was most often the funding agency for the research, necessarily became involved in investigating accusations of abuses or fraud. The complaints covered such matters as abuse of human subjects, credit for authorship of scientific papers, plagiarism, conflicts of interest, and falsification of scientific data. While these were not new phenomena, there were more of them; greater media concentration on such accusations created greater public awareness. Furthermore, since public funds were usually involved, there were congressional inquiries.[31] As a consequence, in 1989 an Office of Scientific Integrity (now entitled Office of Research Integrity) was established within HHS, followed in 2000 by an Office for Human Research Protections.[32] Desiring to avoid HHS action, the Association of American Medical Colleges (AAMC) developed its own set of guidelines proposing that each institution establish a conflict-of-interest committee to review and manage the financial ties of clinical researchers. It was anticipated that these committees would relate closely to the IRBs.

The ethical issues confronting medicine had their impact on almost all health care institutions as well as on medical education. During the nineties virtually every medical school established programs and/or units to teach ethics. The generally elective courses (and, beyond them, lectures, forums, and symposia) were designed not only to sensitize students, but also to probe a range of topics, covering everything from the philosophical roots of ethical behavior to the pragmatic considerations of individual patient care. Notably, the intersection of an aging population with medicine's expanding technological capabilities elevated concerns with issues of death and dying (who shall live and who shall die and, importantly, how they should die). These matters raised important questions that frequently had to be dealt with by the courts. In turn, the courts looked to the medical profession for information and guidance.

The faculty members teaching the medical ethics curriculum came from highly varied backgrounds. While physicians were very much involved, philosophers, clergy, social scientists, historians, and lawyers, among others, also participated. A group of physician-ethicists emerged and created a new area of specialization. Unsurprisingly, a recent survey uncovered that there is no uniformity in the various ethics teaching programs; the authors recommended that basic training in moral reasoning and ethical decision making be integrated both horizontally and vertically in all four years of medical school.[33]

The public's concern with and interest in ethics may in part have been due to an increased suspicion about "experts" (including those in white coats). It could also be attributed to a public recognition that individual behavior by physicians and others was influenced, if not molded, by increasingly complex systems. Finally, we believe it was due to an inherent American ambivalence: respect for the marketplace was inextricably coupled to skepticism about its beneficence. It is as if we believed in market incentives, but were troubled when we learned they had been implemented. This influenced the perception of how ethical issues were resolved in the for-profit sector and of how conflicts of interest could arise in the intersection of new for-profit institutions with a much older not-for-profit sector. It affected "trust."

Over several decades various commissions were appointed to educate both the professional community and the public about ethical issues.[34] Since all phases of medicine and all medical institutions faced such matters, media attention soon followed. Yet it is perhaps the case that the nature of journalism and its emphasis on "the story" were such that there was an emphasis on matters of fraud and abuse to the neglect of more basic questions. Rare were the pieces that asked how to strengthen "professionalism," how systems could be designed to minimize conflicts of interest, how to assure appropriateness of care and interventions, and how to achieve greater equity in the distribution of resources and access to care. Often the latter issues of equity in access to care, in insurance coverage, and more generally in resource allocation were considered "politics" rather than an integral part of the medical ethics discourse. "How to die" seemed to take precedence over "how to live." In this sense, journalists, commissions, and the public mirrored the priorities of medicine: all emphasized the acute rather than the long-term condition.

Medical Education and the Medical Student

Amid the growth in size and complexity of the academic health sciences centers, where was the medical student to be found? Many decades ago medical education (together with the patient care necessary to fulfill that function) had been the central mission of the institution. Now it had become one among any number of activities. The budgets for hospital care (in those institutions where the medical school and the hospital were part of the greater university) dwarfed the budget of the medical school, and often the needs of the hospital (most especially those related to the quest for efficiency and for economies that would end the fiscal year "in the black") took priority. Essential as medical students were, it was also critical that they "not get in the way of the care of the patient" and that they not add time or costs to that care. While there was no deliberate effort to marginalize medical education, the introduction of ever more postgraduate residency training and fellowship programs, along with the emphasis on research, did tend to render the educational mission for the medical student relatively smaller and, perhaps in the eyes of some, less important.

Nevertheless, there were strong counterforces to the marginalization of medical education. First, and perhaps foremost, were the students themselves. Bright, eager, and committed, they competed successfully for admission. The fact that tuitions had increased rapidly and that the students were making substantial economic (and other) sacrifices to attend medical school added legitimacy to their claims on resources and for attention. Their own idealism served as a reminder to medical school administrators and other decision makers that the medical enterprise was about helping others and not simply about money, that medicine was more than just another economic sector or industry. The AAMC, while representing the many interests of the medical schools (serving especially as an advocate for the NIH budget), kept the issues of teaching methods and curriculum very much alive, in keeping with its heritage of annual national teaching institutes dating back to the fifties and sixties.[35] Its yearly meetings and publications (especially the journal *Academic Medicine*) provided for lively exchanges,[36] as did the *Journal of the American Medical Association* (*JAMA*), which had an issue on medical education that appeared every September and (until recently) a monthly section called "MS JAMA," written by and for medical students.[37]

As already noted, the growing complexities of medical care and concern about its quality manifested themselves in the nineties through an emphasis on "evidence-based medicine" spurred by "outcomes research."[38] The close relationship between what was happening in the practice of medicine and what was happening in the education of physicians meant that this focus led to curricular developments in such areas as problem-based learning, clinical reasoning, decision theory, and informatics.

Even so, virtually all medical schools gave continuing attention to the teaching of interviewing skills and the patient-physician relationship. Despite the scientific advances and quantitative methodologies that, along with advanced telecommunications, made it possible to have a protocol for the diagnosis and management of virtually every medical condition, the schools recognized that physician contact with the patient remained the basic component of competent care. While medical educators did not lose sight of this truth, they debated the best way to teach it. Many of them (especially those who were older) remained concerned how, in a world of computer screens, the physician and the patient would continue to relate in a face-to-face manner. That this remained an important issue was clear from the number of patient complaints about failures to make eye contact, the seeming lack of interest on the part of the physician in the social context in which the patient experienced illness, and physician failure to exhibit "caring" characteristics. Educators wondered how and where they could find the time to teach the requisite skills—and, moreover, whether tomorrow's ever more hard-pressed practitioners would be able to find the time to apply what they had been taught.

In an effort to improve the evaluation of student clinical performance, many programs using standardized simulated patients were introduced. Beginning in 2004, in addition to the more traditional assessment of basic knowledge, the standard examinations for medical students included a practical examination to assess their level of clinical expertise.[39] It should come as no surprise that in a society that was becoming accustomed to "virtual" everything, medical education began to think in terms of virtual patients.

It is perhaps useful to remind ourselves that problems in regard to human interaction in the face of technology are not unique to medical education. Similar problems permeate the greater society, as all of us who have spent time pressing buttons on a telephone while vainly hoping to speak to a "live person" can attest. It is not an exaggeration to suggest that the provision of good medical care does require human interaction. Computers, robots, and harried physicians cannot meet the patient's needs for the "caring" function, the function that cannot substitute for, but is as necessary to the practice of good medicine as is the technical expertise that students acquire.

Medical educators have been keenly aware of the obstacles that in recent years have interfered in teaching the priority of the patient-physician relationship: the pressures for more cost-effective care and its constraints on teaching time; the growing numbers of faculty who are pressed to see more patients in ambulatory care settings than in the past; and the greater faculty recognition for research productivity. These trends have, in a cumulative way, eroded the centrality of the teaching and healing mission, and have been referred to as the "hidden curriculum."[40] Furthermore, the students' experiences in the clinic where things move at an increasingly faster pace seem to be at variance with the "academic" lectures about the importance of slowing down in order to get to know and understand the patient. One group of mentors does not appear to practice what another group preaches.

Medical school administrators are increasingly concerned about the quality of teaching, especially given the mounting pressures on the faculty. Basic scientists and clinical researchers need to obtain grant funding for their laboratories, and often to help cover part or all of their salaries; similarly, practicing physicians need to see more patients in order to generate more revenue (for the hospital, if not for the school) to provide their incomes. Indeed, a number of schools claim that they are finding it difficult to recruit physicians who are willing or able to spend time teaching. At least two schools (the University of California at San Francisco and Harvard) have each developed an "academy on medical education" whose faculty members are especially committed to teaching.[41] This represents an effort to introduce a structural component with specific incentives and obligations for the teaching of medical students into the institutional structure of the academic health sciences center.

It is doubtful, however, that this solution, which requires substantial funding since the academy "buys" the faculty member's time, can be generalized. Yet we anticipate that schools facing the problem of faculty recruitment will find their own preferred approaches and will deal with the problem in an effective manner. This view is not based on some irrational optimism, but on our recognition of the resilience of medical education, on its history of adaptation, and on its willingness to change as the external and internal environment changes. We see little reason to suppose that medical schools will abandon that rich history.

Clearly, as an integral part of the medical care sector, medical education is affected by the difficulties confronting the delivery system. Indeed, it is fair to say that in many ways the quality of medical education is held hostage by the dysfunctions in the health care system. More than other parts of the university, the medical school with its clinical teaching and involvement is part of the greater society and cannot stand apart from the world in which it exists. In that important sense it is evident that everyone (patients, students, and faculty) pay a heavy price for the "mess" that the United States health care system, its financing, organization, and increasingly its priorities and values, are experiencing.

Does Medical Education Face a Crisis?

Though it is easy to bewail various constraints and challenges, it is equally clear that, in line with the education system's historical development and traditions, medical educators take their responsibilities to students and to future physicians seriously. Indeed, although educators chronically tend to view medical schools as being in a state of crisis with reference to the educational process, its organization, and financing, there is good reason to question this view.[42] In a recent review of a biography of Abraham Flexner, the historian Janet Tighe wrote, "American Medical schools are in crisis mode. The Association of American Medical Colleges, the schools themselves, such philanthropic entities as the Milbank Foundation, and even the federal government have voiced this opinion. Without denigrating the seriousness of the contemporary situation, it is important to note that we have been here before. The cast of characters has changed, and the financial stakes have increased, but the basic questions are hauntingly similar to ones asked since the early 20th century."[43] The definition of a crisis is "a turning point [for better or for worse] in the course of anything, a decisive or crucial time." Perforce, a situation that appears to be chronic and ever-present should not be considered a "crisis."

This view is documented in an insightful paper by Nicholas Christakis,[44] who reviewed nineteen reports regarding undergraduate medical education published between 1910 and 1993. He found:

Typically, these reports identify strikingly similar problems with medical education, claim that previous reports have gone relatively unheeded, argue that reform is essential and urgent, and prescribe corrections that are also strikingly similar.

The existence of so many similar reports, developed over such a relatively short period raises a perplexing question regarding medical education: either medical schools have remained intractably devoted to deficient modes of education—which seems unlikely, especially given the real changes that have occurred in medical education—or there is another rationale for the promulgation of these reports. In this article, I argue that there is an ethos of reform in US medical education that has two purposes that transcend improving the educational experience of medical students: the reaffirmation of certain core values of the profession and the self-regulation of the profession.

The most recent report on medical education, developed by a committee of ten deans appointed by the AAMC in 2003, seems little different in its assessment than the earlier reports reviewed by Christakis.

However, it does emphasize the problem in clinical education, which "has not kept pace or been responsive enough to shifting patient demographics and desires, changing health system expectations, evolving practice requirements and staffing arrangements, new information, a focus on improving quality, or new technology." The report also takes note of the inroads that managed care has made on clinical training.[45]

Perhaps it is the continued self-critical character of medical educators that contributes to the schools' adaptability and self-renewal. Even as a report of a survey of clinical clerkship directors finds that a majority have negative views of the impact of managed care on teaching,[46] the AAMC Project on the Clinical Education of Medical Students reports,[47]

> There are presently frequent claims from many sources that full-time clinical faculty members do not have time to teach . . . This perception has its roots in the assumption that faculty are hesitant to accept those teaching responsibilities because of the demands placed on their time to conduct research or to provide patient care.
>
> Based on the interviews that were conducted during the school site visits, it is apparent that this perception is inaccurate. Most of the clerkship directors that were interviewed stated that they were able to recruit a sufficient number of qualified faculty to participate in the educational program. Similarly, the medical students that were interviewed reported that they were generally quite satisfied with the amount of time that attending physicians spent with them. In both cases, there was a sense that faculty were willing to commit the time required because many of them enjoy teaching, and decided to pursue an academic career, at least in part, so that they would have opportunities to mentor and teach students.

Medical education can, of course, be improved; certainly there are real problems. We believe that all students would benefit from greater attention to ethical issues involving the distribution of care and issues of conflicts of interest. And we are prepared to argue that all students would gain from a greater understanding of the world in which medicine is practiced and the ways that world is affected by health policy.

We also feel that the welfare of both students and patients would be enhanced were greater attention paid to imparting skills necessary to understand and meet patient needs in a sensitive manner. Finally, as we have heard patient complaints, we cannot help but be struck by the patients' difficulty (particularly in high-powered research environments with their emphasis on subspecialization) in ascertaining who is in charge. It seems more than a pity that while students are told about the importance of teamwork, few seem to realize that the patient needs a team leader to whom he or she can turn.

We would agree with those who argue that in general changes in the health care delivery system have negatively affected medical education. It is true that the expanding emphasis on ambulatory care has had a salutary impact in those geographic areas with managed care entities, hospital-sponsored ambulatory care programs, or strong outpatient departments that are able to organize clinical experiences and monitor the clinical and teaching performance of practicing physicians (as the traditional prepaid group practice could do). However, such organized efforts are scarce. Furthermore, the hospital setting with shorter inpatient stays in which the patient is admitted "at the last minute" and discharged "at the first opportunity" is not conducive to teaching. It is not merely that patients are sicker and that severe time pressures inhibit the orderly teaching process and experience; the patient's progress can hardly be reviewed and fully understood under the prevailing "in-and-out" situation. Nevertheless, since shorter stays are justified on health (as well as economic) grounds, it will be necessary for medical education to adapt to these new conditions.[48]

While the need for improvement cannot be gainsaid, the problems that medical education faces are not so fundamentally ingrained that they require revolutionary structural changes in the curriculum or methods of teaching. It can be argued that just as the major advances in the nation's health came from outside the world of medicine (from actions in the world of public health), so the most important changes in medical education will come from outside the world of the medical school, specifically from changes in the organization and financing of medical care, an area in which most medical educators have continued to show insufficient interest or leadership.

Thus even as we concede the influence of changes in the outside environment and their potential negative impact on medical education, we also believe that many of the changes express themselves through fiscal relationships. And, concomitantly, many of the resulting problems could be addressed with a modest (relative to total national health expenditures) inflow of funds. Whether such funds will be forthcoming hinges on whether society will understand that physicians are a national resource and acts to support the development of that resource.[49]

In large measure medical schools have had no external financial support for their educational function analogous to that provided by the National Institutes of Health for biomedical research. As a consequence students have had to bear a substantial part of those costs through tuition. As costs increased, tuition fees also rose (although there was considerable variation among the schools). State universities and/or universities founded through the federal Morrill Land Grant Act of 1862 tended to have lower tuition rates since they received some support from their respective state governments.[50]

The federal government does provide loan assistance under the Health Professions Educational Assistance Act. In addition, the National Health Service Corps scholarship program, enacted in 1970 and implemented in 1972 when the first twenty clinicians were assigned to medically underserved communities, provides full scholarship support in return for service.[51] Nevertheless, the federal appropriation is quite limited and cannot provide help to all the communities that need it or scholarships to all the students who might choose to join the Corps.

In general medical students have been forced to rely on loans rather than scholarship programs to finance their educations. Scholarship funds were relatively scarce, in part, because the public perception was that physicians had high incomes and therefore could afford to pay off a large educational debt. In 2003 median indebtedness at graduation was $135,000 for graduates of private medical schools and $100,000 for graduates of public medical schools;[52] Congress was not persuaded that this level of indebtedness would have a negative impact on medical practice, specialization, the distribution of physicians (both by specialty and geography), and/or student and physician attitudes. Nor did legislators believe that reduced indebtedness would lead to reductions in physicians' fees. Nevertheless, it is clear that the nation would benefit if graduates were able to enter training and practice less encumbered by debts,[53] and if medical education were financed in a manner that would make that education more accessible to a diverse student body. Regrettably, the question of how best to fund medical education is not an issue that is accorded the priority it warrants.

Already in the late 1980s prospective students were aware of what lay ahead financially. Moreover, they recognized the bureaucratic demands that would be made on them by the increasing corporatization of medical practice. The combination of economic pressures in medicine, the opportunities in other careers, and the growing dissatisfaction within the profession contributed to the decline in applicants to medical school in the mid-nineties, the first such decline since World War II. The hortatory blandishments of faculty members notwithstanding, the students probably had a more accurate and realistic perception of the sociology of future medical practice (at least in the short, and perhaps intermediate, run).

The scientific basis of medicine was exciting, but the prospects for the medical practitioner seemed less so. Articles began to appear in medical journals that spoke to the considerable demoralization of medical practitioners as they faced the twenty-first century.[54] Dr. Fein recalls that at the height of the debate about the Clinton health program he asked the medical students in his course on the financing and organization of medical care to write an essay on the way(s) they believed the Clinton program, if enacted, would affect them. In general they responded that the effects would be felt in two specific ways: (1) they would be pushed into primary care, and (2) they would be employed by for-profit HMOs. While they were troubled by the first prospect, they "accepted" it as meeting national priorities. They were far more concerned about the second, which they believed would restrict their clinical freedom and their ability to serve their patients. They anticipated that they would be "ruled" by managers who would set profits ahead of "good" medical care.

That the external environment makes a difference and that medical schools have changed over the decades are propositions that, as noted earlier, are neither surprising nor disturbing. It is probable that a Dr. Rip Van Winkle who had fallen asleep in the 1940s would hardly recognize the medical school of the early twenty-first century—indeed, he would no doubt be overwhelmed by the differences. The laboratories and the technology would be unfamiliar, the lecture halls would be replete with new and remarkable audiovisual aids, and the observer would be astonished at the versatility (and ubiquitousness) of Power-Point. Nevertheless, it is perhaps the case that nothing would be as astonishing as the changes in the composition of the student body, changes brought about first by the civil rights movement and then by the various pressures for diversity. Stimulated by the transformations in the greater society and assisted by antidiscrimination legislation, the AAMC and a number of the individual schools developed explicit efforts to recruit more minority and female medical students. This effort has largely been successful in respect to gender distribution: recent entering classes have approximately equal numbers of men and women.

This recruitment has proven more difficult in regard to minorities, perhaps because of prevailing income disparities, the educational disadvantages in earlier schooling faced by many minority applicants, fewer visible role models, and/or the competition from other professional disciplines such as law and business administration. The continuing battle in and around the issue of affirmative action (even after the Bakke case and the more recent Supreme Court action in 2003 partially validating University of Michigan admission policies designed to create a more diverse student body) has not made the task facing the universities and their medical schools any easier. The fact that there are no easy answers to these issues (which have a very long history) should not be taken as license to shy away from the hard ones. "No easy answer" is not a synonym for "let's give up." Rather, it just means "we must be more imaginative and try even harder."

As the twentieth century drew to a close, concerns about the numbers of physicians available to care for an expanding population resurfaced. The 1981 projections by the Graduate Medical Education National Advisory Committee (GMENAC) that there would be a large oversupply of physicians by the year 2000 were not borne out.[55] More recently one group of observers has estimated physician need by relating the demand for physician services to the growth in population and in GDP, and has projected a need for 5,000 additional graduates per year. In turn, this would require twenty-five new medical schools.[56] Other observers have called for a significant expansion in medical school capacity because the number of international medical graduates who are required to fill first-year residency positions impinges negatively on the medical care in the nations from which they come.[57] That argument is reinforced by the consideration that such expansion would accommodate the approximately 5,000 United States citizens annually enrolling in foreign medical schools.

As already discussed, the history of projections of physician supply and demand suggests that it is difficult to reach consensus on these matters. Therefore, it should not come as a surprise to discover that still other observers discern no significant current or prospective shortage in physician supply. Furthermore, these observers believe that the medical care delivery system exhibits a considerable adaptability and elasticity. They remind us that nonphysicians (nurse-practitioners and physician assistants) also deliver medical care services,[58] that new technologies can affect (and perhaps reduce) the need for physicians' services, and that the reliance on international medical graduates provides a safety valve that makes it less important to have a definitive policy on "how many are enough." In an effort to resolve conflicting views on the "shortage" issue, the AAMC announced the establishment in December 2003 of a new unit to study physician supply.[59]

We believe that in light of current state budgetary problems, the costs that would need to be incurred in establishing new medical schools make it unlikely that a solution to any shortfall in the future supply of physicians and of physician services lies in opening additional schools. Existing schools may be able to increase enrollment, but any such increases will probably be marginal. America's needs will more plausibly be met by continuing to rework the structure and organization of the delivery system (that is, what is done, where it is done, and by whom it is done) and moreover by attracting graduates of foreign schools. The conclusion that there seems to be little "excess capacity" in the existing medical education institutions system and that the prospect of building new medical schools is dim, encourages (indeed, forces) us to consider the ways in which the existing system can provide more services and the degree to which services now provided are necessary. In turn, this forces a reassessment of the roles played by the various kinds of personnel and whether those roles can be modified in an appropriate manner.

Finally, it is important to note that there is little reason to believe that an increase in the number of physicians would address the important and persistent issues involving uneven distribution of clinicians by geography and specialty. There are too few physicians in many parts of our nation, just as there are too few physicians who provide primary care and family practice services. Yet the needs of rural and inner-city areas, exacerbated by the shortage of physicians who would provide primary care services to our low-income and minority neighbors, are not likely to be met by a strategy that simply increases the total number of physicians and floods the system. Rather, they must be met by recalling and reinvigorating earlier efforts that developed and supported neighborhood and community health centers. Those centers were able to attract physicians and thus contributed to the redeployment of the physician workforce. Again, as in so many other areas, we conclude that the problems we face cannot be solved by individual physicians, but instead require system change.

Most of the major changes in the delivery of health care services during the twentieth century have been incremental. Nevertheless, there were exceptions, born out of a sense of general crisis. The first such exception was the response to the Great Depression of the 1930s. Another set of major policy changes arose in response to the civil rights revolution and the War on Poverty of the mid-sixties during the early years of President Lyndon Baines Johnson's administration.

Perhaps the nature of our politics is such that the nation will be forced to wait for another crisis that will serve as a stimulus for substantial reform. It could be that the continuing and rapid increase in health expenditures and health insurance premiums and the mounting cost of prescription drugs will be sufficient to shape a kind of health crisis atmosphere. The continuing inequities in care, and the growing dissatisfaction of the public and clinicians with the complexities each confronts, might also feed a sense of societal anxiety. Or the threat of bioterrorism may serve to focus attention on the need for a sound public health infrastructure and thus for renewed government support for public health. Perhaps we are approaching a time when more systemic changes will indeed be considered. Yet we recognize that there appears to be a large gap between current dissatisfaction and the willingness to call for and take action. It is quite possible that concern and inaction (even complacency) are not mutually exclusive conditions.

We return to the model that we articulated earlier: the need for a knowledge base, a social strategy, and political will. Our concluding chapters will summarize our views and offer a social strategy for change, perhaps one that might contribute to creating a climate in which the political will to move the health care system forward can be galvanized.

Part IV

ANTICIPATING THE NEXT
REVOLUTION (2005 AND BEYOND)

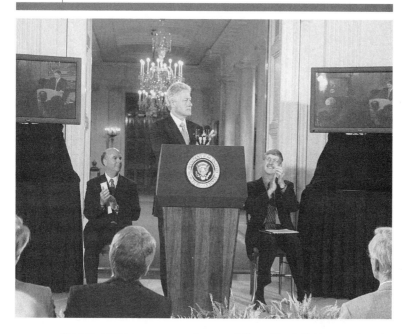

President Clinton announces the completion of the initial sequencing of
the human genome on June 26, 2000—one of the great events in the
history of science. With the President are Francis Collins, Director of the
National Human Genome Research Institute *(right)* and Craig Venter,
President and Chief Scientific Officer, Celera Genomics Corporation *(left)*.
Photograph © Ron Sachs/CNP/CORBIS.

7 | Medical Challenges and Opportunities

In these, our concluding chapters, we look to the future. None of us know precisely how the United States will change during the twenty-first century, the "values" that will impel us in the years ahead, the shape of our international relations, the size and nature of our economy, the structure of our society, the particular ways in which medicine will evolve, and what "revolutions" will occur. Nevertheless, we do know that today's health care system, the manner in which it is organized, its level of funding, and the ways that health services are financed for and by our population are not meeting our nation's requirements. This is true even after more than a decade of an experiment in free-market dominance and a reliance on competitive forces. The gap between today's health care system's potential contributions and actual performance is great. It will grow even wider if beneficial health care interventions continue to emanate from our laboratories only to encounter a health care system that is unable or unwilling to meet the challenge of delivering these new interventions to all of the populations in need.

Although we do not know the speed with which the nation will develop new approaches to health care delivery and new patterns of organization and financing, we do know that neither the timing nor the nature of the various changes is either preordained or determined by some random roll of the dice. Whatever occurs will be heavily dependent on the choices that our nation makes at various decision opportunities. Those choices will be shaped by experience, culture, values, and politics, matters on which many Americans whose histories are different disagree. Nevertheless, we believe (and this belief is sustained by historical experience and by faith in our democracy) that the debates in which we shall engage can alter attitudes. We offer these final comments with the hope that they will contribute to making those debates richer and more thoughtful than they otherwise might be. We do so with full recognition that there are many important health care topics that we do not discuss. The fact that a reader's favorite issue is referred to very briefly or perhaps even entirely omitted, should not suggest it is insignificant. Rather, it is a reminder that the health care field is exceedingly rich and complex and that we have elected to focus our attention on medical care and medical education, only two among many important subsets of that entire field.

We begin this chapter with a discussion of some of the challenges and opportunities that clinical medicine faces both in the United States and in the developing nations at the beginning of the twenty-first century. Because meeting those challenges will require resources, in the next sections of the chapter we review the supply of physicians, medical education, and various issues involving medical research. A third section moves to an examination of the manner in which these resources are organized, and deals with the ways by which the effectiveness and efficiency of the delivery system might be enhanced.

Nevertheless, it is clear that even if our science base, therapeutic advances, physicians, other health care workers, and institutional infrastructure are all sufficient, health care needs will not be met unless our nation becomes deeply committed to equity as an operational concept and finds a better method to make effective health care available to all its population. The final chapter will discuss the need for a universal insurance program, and the issues that must be resolved in designing such a plan, and will then offer a series of suggestions about ways to proceed that would address some of the concerns that have divided policy makers.

Health in the Twenty-First Century

The twentieth century witnessed the decline of infectious diseases in the developed world. Yet, even as some observers dared to suggest that such diseases would soon be eliminated, a new infectious disease, the human immunodeficiency virus (HIV), emerged. The consequence of the infection was acquired immune deficiency disease (AIDS), which has resulted in millions of deaths in countries all over the world. It is estimated that at the present time 42 million persons worldwide are infected, 30 million of them in Africa.

The infection, which can be acquired through body fluids (often by exposure through sexual contact, sharing of contaminated needles, or blood transfusions from infected donors), may not cause symptoms for months or years. It is clear that preventive measures require public education and changes in the behavior of populations, especially sexual behavior and intravenous drug use. Hence the quest for more effective preventive measures, such as vaccines, is being pursued. In the interim improved therapies are becoming available, though they are both costly and cumbersome. AIDS is and will remain a severe threat to the health of the populations and to the economies of major parts of the world.

Because they compromise the immune system, HIV infections have also facilitated the reemergence of tuberculosis and other opportunistic infections as major health concerns globally. Unfortunately, multidrug resistance to tuberculosis has developed, making it more difficult to treat.[1] The World Health Organization (WHO) is developing strategies for better control, but it is clear that in many parts of the world (and in places with a high population density, such as prisons) the successful implementation of such strategies will pose a major challenge.

A third large-scale infectious disease, malaria, continues to be a serious public health problem in the developing world. Since its epidemiology has long been known, it had been expected that malaria by now would be better managed, particularly through mosquito control. Even though this objective has been high on the agenda of the WHO for many years, the complexity and cost of the necessary measures have impeded progress. Efforts to develop an effective vaccine have thus far not proven successful, although there are recent promising developments.

In addition to the infectious diseases cited thus far, war and particularly its aftereffects in their own right create significant health problems in many parts of the world. The developing world, roiled by conflict, often faces additional burdens of disease resulting from the absence of clean water supplies and from shortfalls in sanitation, hygiene, and immunizations. All these serve to keep infectious diseases high on the health agendas of these countries.

In the more affluent countries, in the latter half of the twentieth century the focus shifted from infectious diseases (with the exception of HIV) to diseases that are multifactorial in origin. Analysis indicates that a significant decline in mortality from cardiovascular diseases such as heart disease and stroke began in the United States at about the time of the first Surgeon-General's Advisory Committee Report on Smoking and Health in 1964, due in part to the resulting decrease in cigarette smoking. The improved mortality rate also followed on significant advances in the development of effective pharmacological agents to control high blood pressure. Nor should we ignore the fact that individuals have become more aware of the need for exercise, better dietary practices, and the importance of detection and control of high blood pressure, and that many of them have acted upon that newfound knowledge.

Conversely, the prevention of cancer has proven to be a much more difficult challenge. The reduction in cigarette smoking has resulted in some reduction in mortality from lung cancer among men. This success story (and it is by no means a complete success) has not been fully matched for other cancer sites. We continue to need more research on cancer causation and prevention that would enable us to deal more effectively with the many varieties of cancer. Although it is decades since President Nixon proclaimed a "war on cancer," progress has been slow. There have been a number of advances and a greater ability to treat a variety of cancers, but we cannot yet claim to have had a major impact on overall measures of health.

Often neglected in public health considerations are issues concerning mental health. Analysis undertaken by the World Health Organization has documented that mental health concerns, especially depression, are major factors in morbidity and disability. It is estimated that by 2020 depression will be the most frequent cause of disability. Fortunately, the advances in research in the neurosciences and a better understanding of mental processes make it possible to mount more effective preventive and therapeutic programs.[2] Nevertheless, there is a major "disconnect" between the needs and the resources available.

One of the most important issues facing all societies is fostering the optimal development of young children in order to facilitate their learning as they enter the school years. Abundant evidence exists to demonstrate that children growing up in environments of poverty often are at a disadvantage in learning.[3] Programs that incorporate stimulating early child care (including comprehensive health services) can be important in overcoming such disadvantages. Even though difficult to quantify, the failure to support early child care adequately may result in the greatest loss of human potential.

Although literacy on health issues, including nutritional issues, has increased over the years, a gradual population shift toward the overweight and the obese has occurred. In 1999–2000 over 30 percent of the adult United States population was classified as obese and 64 percent was classified as obese or overweight.[4] Since overweight persons are at higher risk for a number of health problems, especially Type II diabetes, these numbers are more than merely disconcerting or esthetically displeasing. According to a RAND Corporation study, if obesity continues to increase at its current rate in the United States, by 2020 about one in five health care dollars spent on persons ages 50–69 could be consumed by obesity-related medical problems, a rise of about 50 percent from 2000.[5] This may also reverse some of the gains that had been made in reducing mortality from cardiovascular diseases. It should be clear that public health education alone will not be sufficient to stem what has become an epidemic. We will also need programs that motivate people to act on the knowledge they have. We require not only an effective social strategy but also the political will to implement that strategy (even in the face of opposition from segments of the food industry).

The Expanding Science Base

This roster of concerns and problems should be counterbalanced with a brief review of the expanding science base and thus the possible advances that may help address the challenges we confront. It is important to understand that at no time in the history of medicine have there been such clear grounds for optimism about medical progress, though the advances we foresee may not take place tomorrow or in a year or even in a decade. Nor do we wish to imply that, having made great discoveries and developed therapies based on the new knowledge, we will have the strategies and political consensus in place to make them available to all the population. But we do want to make clear that the problems we have listed are likely to become less vexing, and potentially surmountable.

(1) Advances in molecular biology and human genetics have made it possible to map and sequence the entire human genome. Although some in the scientific community thought that an all-out effort to accomplish this goal was not urgent, the advocates won out. In 1993 the National Institutes of Health began such an effort by bringing together an international consortium of universities and other not-for-profit and public research centers. This endeavor was paralleled by that of the publicly traded for-profit Celera Corporation, whose leadership believed that private enterprise could complete the task sooner. Both the NIH-sponsored group, the International Genome Sequencing Consortium, whose findings were open to all (including the private group) and made available on a continuing basis, as well as Celera (which chose not to make its findings public), completed the task at about the same time in 2001.[6] Having determined that sequencing organisms was not a profitable business model, Celera, as part of a larger company, moved on to different pursuits. The NIH continues to believe that the sequencing of other organisms is important to the understanding of the biological mechanisms of human disease (as well as of potential bioterrorism agents) and therefore supports a small number of very large-scale not-for-profit sequencing centers.

Basic advances in genetics provide a better understanding of how heredity interacts with environment to produce diseases, and there are great expectations for the practical applications of such knowledge. The knowledge acquired thus far has led to screening tests for a number of inborn errors of metabolism (such as newborn screening for phenylketonuria and for some twenty other genetic disorders)[7] and to prenatal diagnosis for several additional disorders. Thus far, however, few treatments have been developed. Further scientific advances will be required to develop effective preventive, diagnostic, and therapeutic techniques. The "new genetics" raises important issues of costs and of privacy. The former include the question whether the therapeutic benefits of genetic knowledge will be covered by insurance and by Medicare and Medicaid (or, for example, will be considered "experimental"). Will these new therapies, whose discovery is, at least in part, made possible by taxpayers' dollars, be within the reach of the general population, that is, of those very taxpayers? The issue of privacy is also important (and not unrelated to the issue of insurance and therefore of costs to the individual). It seems clear that if insurers (or employers) know enough about an individual's genes (the ultimate "preexisting condition"), they may discriminate against those individuals who they believe will be at high risk of incurring above-average costs. To a significant degree the American health insurance system has been based upon the sharing of risk (though, unfortunately, on less than a universal basis). That system may fall apart in the face of the new knowledge that genetics may bring. That will be especially so if the movement to individual medical savings accounts (made possible in recent Medicare reform legislation and applicable to the entire population) grows and brings further fragmentation to the insurance market, and as a result individuals with the "proper" genes (and others who believe they are of low risk) leave the general insurance pool.

(2) A much greater understanding of immunology has had sweeping effects on clinical practice. A cluster of diseases came to be known as autoimmune disorders: rheumatoid arthritis, lupus erythematosus, ulcerative colitis, and Crohn's disease, among others. These were subjected to reinvigorated efforts at improved diagnoses and treatments, and as a consequence of new drug therapies, the care and the outlook for patients have improved.

The deepening knowledge of immunology was perhaps most evident from the role it played in facilitating organ transplantation. It is obvious that immunologic compatibility is a key factor in the success of this surgery. Indeed, the first successful organ transplantation of a kidney in 1954,[8] a truly pioneering venture in surgical technology, was equally pioneering in choosing an identical twin as the donor (a clear recognition of the problems of immunologic rejection). Immunosuppressive drugs became a key factor in extending transplantation to other organs such as the heart, liver, and lungs. It is conceivable that a successful transplantation of islet cells of the pancreas may ultimately transform the management of Type I diabetes.

(3) Research in the neurosciences has grown rapidly in recent decades. The nineties were declared "the decade of the brain,"[9] and much of the promise was fulfilled. Perhaps no professional research society grew as rapidly as the Society for Neuroscience, whose membership exploded from approximately 500 in 1970 to over 34,000 today.[10] The basic scientific advances led in many directions. Efforts begun in the 1980s have since identified the mutant genes implicated in over fifty disorders of the nervous system, including Huntington's disease, Friedreich's ataxia, some of the muscular dystrophies, and familial early-onset Alzheimer's disease.[11] Although clinical applications have not yet developed, there is hope that the better understanding of these disease processes will lead to improved prevention as well as treatment. Though there have been gains in studying the neurochemistry of Parkinson's disease and some therapeutic applications have been encouraging, much more knowledge is needed for successful treatment.

As noted earlier, the interaction of genetics (nature) with environment (nurture) in early development has received much attention in recent years, including from this field of medical investigation. Through new neuroimaging and neurochemistry studies, scientists have a better understanding of how impoverished environments affect the developing brain of the infant and young child.[12] Furthermore, the growing knowledge and understanding about the mechanisms by which messages are transmitted in the central nervous system have given rise to significant improvement in the treatment for a variety of mental disorders. The field of neurochemistry has led to medications for bipolar disorder, manic-depressive psychosis, depression, schizophrenia, Tourette's syndrome, and others, thereby transforming the practice of psychiatry.

As longevity has increased, more attention has been devoted to brain changes associated with aging. Growing concerns about mental decline, particularly Alzheimer's disease, have generated research that provides a better understanding of biochemical and structural modifications that occur with these disorders. In turn, there are expectations that this new knowledge will lead to better outcomes.

And the outlook for groups with other afflictions shows similar promise. For example, people with sensory impairments, particularly of vision and hearing, are benefiting from efforts to prevent or treat loss of function through such developments as cochlear implants for hearing loss. That said, as with other already enumerated conditions, many unresolved problems that require more research still remain.

(4) Advances in technology, including imaging techniques, have done much to improve diagnostic processes and treatment, and merit specific comment. Computerized axial tomography (CAT) scans and magnetic resonance imaging (MRI) provide much clearer images than conventional x-rays and can be combined with biochemical markers for more refined diagnostic and possibly therapeutic targeting. The noninvasive nature and greater accuracy of these methods have rendered various invasive imaging procedures obsolete. Improved visualization methods also have made possible a number of surgical innovations. Thus arthroscopic visualization and surgery of various joints have become routine, as has laparoscopic surgery.

Furthermore, the new technologies, including more tissue-compatible materials, have enabled the replacement of joints (such as hip and knee and, less frequently, ankle), of cataracts by lenses, and of heart valves as well as blood vessels. The world of medicine is surely one that even the most incurable optimist could not have imagined fifty years ago.

(5) Research on cells (stem cells) obtained from an in-vitro fertilized egg (blastocyst) that is intended to be discarded has determined that these cells have the potentiality (hence pluripotency) to develop into various tissues of the body. Further stem-cell research is expected to open up great possibilities for treatment of diabetes, Parkinson's, Alzheimer's, and many other diseases.

Since these cells initially have embryonic origins, the issue of when life begins has become significant in public policy discussions concerning continuing support for such research. Those who oppose abortion equate use of these embryonic tissues with the termination of life even though these embryos would otherwise be discarded. As a consequence of its support for this position, the Bush administration limited federal funding only to research that used stem cells already available to research workers as of August 9, 2001. This has left research workers in the United States (though, of course, not in other nations) with more limited stem-cell access if they pursue federal funding. As a result of an initiative that received popular support, the state of California will make public funding available for such research. It seems clear that other states may follow. New research possibilities would also be opened if cells carrying a genetic defect could be cloned and introduced into an ovum, thereby providing opportunities to learn much more about the development of disease processes.

Although there will be continuing debate about the propriety of carrying on such research, the work will go forward, particularly in those countries where these issues are not so politicized. Given the magnitude of the scientific possibilities, pragmatism is likely to prevail in bringing the potential benefits of such research to clinical care.

(6) The application of advances in new communication technologies has been significant not only in improving medical care but also in the emergence of the medical Internet. Electronic access via a desktop computer to medical libraries, journals, and colleagues, as well as to medical records, is transforming practice. The development of increasingly effective protocols for diagnostic and therapeutic management of patients is made possible by applying these technologies.

Concomitant with the use of the new communications technology by health professionals has been the computer's role in empowering consumers to be more proactive in discussions with their physicians and other care providers and to make more knowledgeable choices about health care. The ubiquity of the medical Internet now makes it possible for individuals to become more engaged in self-care while becoming better equipped to use medical care in more informed ways.

The last decade has witnessed the emergence of the field of "health literacy," which the Institute of Medicine (IOM) has defined as the "degree to which individuals can obtain, process, and understand the basic health information and services they need to make appropriate health decisions."[13] Studies indicate that people with low health literacy understand health information less well, receive less preventive health care, and use more costly health services (such as emergency department services) more frequently. It is clear that language differences and cultural issues are important considerations in formulating effective programs for health literacy. The IOM has made comprehensive programmatic recommendations for continuing national efforts to promote a health-literate America.

(7) The quantitative sciences, particularly epidemiology and biostatistics, have facilitated much of the research on which clinical improvements have been based. In the days when we had few diagnostic and therapeutic interventions, in the days before computers, these methods were not nearly as useful. But with the advent of new diagnostic tools and the burgeoning of new drugs that require careful evaluation of effectiveness and efficiency, these methods are critically important.

The basic contributions of these sciences to the study of populations have been key to our identification of new diseases, the examination of patterns of distribution of diseases in populations, the improvement of preventive practices, the assessment of effective screening methods for early detection of disease, and, more recently, a greater understanding of which health-promoting practices are effective. The evaluation of therapeutic agents has, appropriately, come to rely on randomized clinical trials.

The advances in public health and the greater capacity of schools of public health to apply epidemiology and biostatistics to population-based studies have stimulated and enabled a paradigm shift. While the earlier emphasis on disease prevention has not become obsolete, a new emphasis seems timely: that of health promotion. Conceptually this represents a shift from a focus on defining health as the absence of disease to one that cultivates a positive concentration on health and, therefore, the development of strategies to promote optimal health (difficult as that may be to define).

While medical schools are heavily and appropriately focused on clinical care, schools of public health have assumed a leadership role in providing the intellectual infrastructure for setting public health priorities, practices, and education. These developments made it possible for the then-Surgeon-General, Dr. David Satcher, to set public health goals in 2000 for the year 2010, and to introduce a creative approach to the campaign to improve the public's health. He especially emphasized the importance of reducing disparities in morbidity and mortality among population groups.

Recent data bear out his concern. For example, while the white infant mortality rate in the United States in 2001 was 5.7 deaths per 1,000 live births, the rate for African Americans was over twice as high, at 13.3.[14] Similarly, 302 per 100,000 white American men die of heart disease, while this is true for 385 per 100,000 African-American males.[15] Furthermore, though considerable attention has been devoted to ethnic disparities, Dr. Satcher noted that other disparities, such as those associated with economic, geographic, and occupational conditions, also are significant. These gaps are accentuated by a lower quality of health services for minority populations. A recent report indicates that physicians who served the black population were less likely to be board-certified, and reported that African Americans had less access to high-quality subspecialists, diagnostic imaging, or nonemergency room hospital care.[16]

The approach exemplified in Satcher's goals is designed to raise health levels among groups with the lowest records and outlook and thus reduce inequalities and improve the nation's health as a whole. This strategy can be applied at all levels: internationally, nationally, and within states and localities. But to do so clearly requires better data, more sophisticated analyses, sound social strategies, and, as always, the political will to meet these challenges. The role of schools of public health in undertaking this work and in training scholars and researchers to assist in these efforts will be central to their success.

Physician Work Issues

As we have indicated, the analysis of physician supply has been fraught with difficulties. As a consequence of the major problems in workforce analysis, there has been a continuing lively debate among those who study issues and policies concerning the total number of physicians and those in the various specialties. This debate has been useful, since, among other things, it reminds us that a focus on needed physician supply is much too narrow an orientation. We must also account for the wide geographical variation in the utilization of services within the United States, as is illustrated in the studies by John Wennberg and his colleagues.[17] How does one go about determining how many physicians a nation "needs," given the variations in utilization? (For example, in 1996 visits to physicians by Medicare beneficiaries in the last six months of life exhibited regional variations by as much as a factor of 5.6.) In considering the supply of physicians it is imperative to ask what physicians do, whether those tasks need doing, and whether they need to be done by physicians.

Yet even those questions would be insufficient. A newly trained physician will spend many years in practice in a field that surely will not remain static. Thus a major problem in quantifying future need and demand for physicians relates to the potential impacts of applying our rapidly developing new knowledge. While one might assume that the expanding knowledge base renders medical care more complex, the opposite may also be true, that is, that medical care may be rendered simpler. An obvious example involves the remarkable decline in the infectious diseases over the last century. One of this book's co-authors, during a pediatric residency just prior to World War II, spent more than half his time caring for children with acute infectious diseases that American medical students educated today will never see. We can take note that over the same time period nutritional deficiency disorders such as rickets and scurvy have virtually disappeared. Thus much physician time was saved and that which was "banked" could be drawn upon to deal with other child health problems such as developmental disabilities. Robert Haggerty defined these conditions as the "new morbidity."[18] It is clear that we lack an agreed-upon methodology by which to estimate the contribution of scientific advances, or to assess the need for physician services (let alone for physicians), or to evaluate alternate ways to assure that those needs can be met.

Although the long period of graduate medical education should have rendered undergraduate medical education more flexible, that flexibility was slow in coming. The rationalization that medical education had to cope with the vast expansion in knowledge was sometimes used to counter the common criticism that the faculty tried to incorporate too much material in teaching in the classroom and at the patient's bedside. But this may have been a fallacious argument. More knowledge does not necessarily make teaching more difficult. We should remember J. Robert Oppenheimer's observation: "On the other hand, there is a more encouraging aspect of . . . scientific knowledge. As it grows, things, in some ways, get much simpler. They do not get simpler because one discovers a few fundamental principles which the man in the street can understand and from which he can derive everything else. But we do find an enormous amount of order. The world is not random and whatever order it has seems in large part 'fit,' as Thomas Jefferson said, for the human intelligence. The enormous variety of facts yields to some kind of arrangement, simplicity, generalization."[19]

One can conclude that, viewed pragmatically, over the last century the supply of physicians has turned out to be reasonably adequate. It is certainly true that patients and potential patients are "unhappy" and angered by the complexities of the medical care system. Some of the public's reaction may be a function of the difficulty with which they gain entry into the system (for example, the ease or difficulty in making an appointment and the waiting time before appointments in certain specialties), but the issue is largely one of maldistribution (by specialty and location) rather than of total supply. In largest measure, patient unhappiness stems from factors exogenous to the total number of physicians.

While, in general, the part of the population that is affluent and has health insurance coverage tends to be relatively well served, that part of the population with lower income and with less or no insurance does have real access problems. Nevertheless, it is not clear that these problems stem from an overall shortage of physicians or that they would be addressed by increasing their number. If the United States adopts a universal insurance program (or if the nation were to develop mechanisms to attain a more equitable income distribution that would enable more persons to enter the medical marketplace), it might be advisable to increase the total number of physicians. Nevertheless, we believe it is necessary to add a cautionary note: we dare not assume that increases in the supply of physicians (a not inexpensive proposition) will attract physicians to serve those populations most in need or in those geographic areas with the largest shortages.

Nor can we be assured that an increase in the number of physicians would "solve" the problem of the distribution of practitioners in the various medical specialties. Flooding the system would undoubtedly lead to higher costs and might lead to lower quality of care as a result of greater utilization of procedures that are unnecessary or of only marginal benefit. That would be an unnecessary price to pay to achieve the necessary redistribution of personnel and of services. Put simply, we believe that maldistribution issues are best addressed through emphasizing support for community health centers, other forms of organized practice, an expansion of the National Health Service Corps, rationalization of medical tasks, appropriate incentives, and such other actions as address the specific problem (often of a local nature).[20]

In any event, it is clear that, given the highly decentralized private and public medical education system and the innumerable unknowns (including the growing importance of pharmaceuticals and of genetics), that more precise needs assessments are not possible. Furthermore, even if they were possible and we reached agreement on the numbers, it is doubtful that such agreement could lead to appropriate actions in a sector that is decentralized, where the loci for decisions on education, specialization, and location are diffused. It seems more certain that the health care system is quite adaptable and can operate successfully with different physician-population ratios.

The context of medical education also has changed significantly over the century. Initially, medical school was the terminal education of the physician; gradually the one year of internship became a requirement for licensure, and still later specialized training beyond the internship became the pattern. The transformation of the post-medical school training period was embraced because of the consensus that increases in medical knowledge and advances in technology made longer educational preparation necessary. As a consequence there was virtually no resistance to this prolongation, even in spite of the indebtedness of many medical students.

As levels of indebtedness have grown to today's much higher levels, so, too, have the levels of anxiety about the high costs of becoming a physician and the years of training required to do so. It is perhaps also the case that as the health sector has become more commercial and as the number of articles, symposia, forums, and lectures that deal with the economics of the health sector have expanded, residents in training have become increasingly aware of and concerned about their status in this sector and what they may view as exploitation. Perhaps they feel that their own "bottom lines" are as important as those of the institutions in which they are being trained; perhaps they feel that the institutions are addressing their budgetary concerns by using collusive anticompetitive behavior to keep resident salaries relatively low. Surely, they are aware that they work hard and that their contributions to the care of patients would command higher rates of compensation in the open market for physician services.

There is increasing recognition of the ambiguity surrounding the role of residents: are they students or are they employees? As part of the current questioning of traditional practices (and also in keeping with the increased concern about quality of care), new standards for maximum hours of work by residents in defined time periods have been adopted. Some residents went so far as to file an antitrust suit against the National Resident Matching Program (NRMP), "the matchmaker" for the residency selection process (which, when adopted in 1952, had been regarded as a progressive move designed to bring order out of the chaos that then governed the process). They charged that the NRMP involved anticompetitive behavior by hospitals, behavior that served to keep salaries low and working conditions long and arduous, the classic characteristics of an exploitive situation. In April 2004 Congress enacted legislation that stated that the use of the NRMP did not violate antitrust law. On this basis the original suit was dismissed.[21]

As we have noted, it is our belief that the self-conscious concern that medical school faculty members exhibit about the quality of medical education generates tensions that on the whole have had a favorable effect. Judged by any conventional criteria, students perform well.

They appear to arrive at their graduate medical education programs well prepared for the next phase of learning patient care and skills. The fact that students achieve a basic educational competence (especially when we consider the heterogeneity of the schools they attend) is a remarkable achievement for a country so large and diverse. There always is room for improvement and, as already discussed, we do recognize some specific shortcomings. Nevertheless, we do not view medical education with the same degree of alarm as do some others.[22]

We believe that medical education is remarkably resilient and that many of the problems it faces arise from forces outside the educational institutions. Thus they will not be solved by "reforming" medical education since they derive from an exogenously determined medical care financing system that, among other things, presses in upon faculty and potential faculty and forces them to devote an inordinate proportion of time to generating income through research grants or patient care,[23] and thus allowing less time to devote to creating tomorrow's physicians. Our medical students will be equipped with the necessary knowledge base in science and medicine. The greater problems they will face will be those involving the financing and organization of services. Regrettably, preparation on these matters (as is also true about ethics and public policy) tends to be neglected.

The resilience of medical education is all the more remarkable, since, as we have noted, in contrast to research it has not had a clear and consistent funding pattern. Shortly after World War II the research leadership in the United States arrived at a partnership with government that provided significant federal funding for medical research and much public participation in its policy making. There has been no comparable federal support for medical education—except for programs to increase the numbers of physicians. This latter emphasis has been understandable since physicians, like other Americans, are mobile, and achieving an adequate physician supply is a national issue. Nevertheless, at various times it has been suggested that federal funds be made available to provide more broadly focused, firm, and continuing support for medical education. Clearly, the sums involved (relative to the health funding commitments the federal budget now entails) would not represent a burden of "break the bank" proportions.

Funds could be allocated on a per student basis even as the individual characteristics of medical schools would continue to be honored. The regional subcommissions and the national commission that we shall propose (and discuss in the next chapter) as mechanisms to help rationalize money flows and resources could play a central role in organizing the system of universal insurance and in the establishment of planning mechanisms. They could also serve a key function in helping the various regions meet their needs through fine-tuning educational allocations that are responsive to the unique health problems of a specific region.[24]

No discussion of physicians and physician supply would be complete without comment on two additional matters. Both have an impact on the environment within which physicians practice and therefore on the environment within which patients receive care. The first matter deals with the "malpractice crisis."[25] The second concerns the American Medical Association (AMA) and its role as the public voice of American medicine. It is to these we now turn.

Malpractice Insurance

As the new century came into being, physicians were angered by what they saw as a buildup in administrative burdens and interference by third-party payers. In addition, many physicians concluded that they had to work harder to maintain their income, and others found that, even when they increased their workload, their net income declined. The media and professional journals were reporting exciting scientific advances, but day-to-day practice was becoming less rewarding. Superimposed on this unhappiness, if not malaise, was the fact that physicians in a number of states (Pennsylvania, West Virginia, and New Jersey, for example) faced very large jumps in malpractice insurance premiums and in some instances the withdrawal of insurers from the market, and that physicians in other states were concerned that, sooner or later, they too would find it difficult to obtain and/or pay for insurance.

Physicians further complained that they were being harassed by malpractice claims (including claims that did not result in litigation) and sometimes found that their insurer settled claims that individual physicians felt were without merit. As they saw it, such settlements harmed a physician's reputation and record, and though there may have been a prior agreement in the insurance contract permitting the insurer to make such settlements, the physician was angered that he or she had no control in the matter. Many physicians reported that they were caught between HMOs and other medical care insurers who, on the one hand, wanted to hold premiums down and therefore pressured physicians to "do less" and the need, on the other hand, to "do more"—that is, to practice defensive medicine in order to reduce claims and litigation and, failing that, to be able to erect a defense against such claims should they arise. These additional interventions add undetermined costs to the American health care system.

The AMA defines a state as in a "liability crisis" if patients have less access to care from doctors in certain specialties because high malpractice insurance premiums have driven physicians to retire earlier, move to other jurisdictions, change their specialization, or otherwise withdraw their services. The AMA concluded that as of June 2004 twenty states were in that category.[26] In early 2003 physicians in some states engaged in "strikes" to protest their plight and pressed public officials to impose upper limits ("caps") on the pain and suffering portion of malpractice judgments and/or to limit attorney compensation. In the spring of 2004 there were reports that some physicians were refusing medical treatment to lawyers, their families, and their employees except in emergencies. There also were reports that specific hospitals had prohibited staff members from testifying on behalf of patients (while permitting them to appear on behalf of physicians and hospitals).[27]

Few things in medicine and its infrastructure are quite as simple as might first appear. That is certainly the case with the "malpractice crisis." It is a fact that in some geographic areas and for some specialties malpractice insurance rates have increased rapidly over the last few years and far more rapidly than the fees that physicians receive from patients or through insurance, Medicare, or Medicaid. The Government Accountability—previously "Accounting"—Office (GAO) studied seven states in depth and concluded that there was considerable variation in the level and movement of premiums. The GAO report notes that "the largest writer of medical malpractice insurance in Florida increased premium rates for general surgeons in Dade County by approximately 75 percent from 1999 to 2000, while the largest insurer in Minnesota increased premium rates for the same specialty by about 2 percent over the same period. The resulting 2002 premium rate quoted by the insurer in Florida was $174,300 a year, more than 17 times the $10,140 premium rate quoted by the insurer in Minnesota." Furthermore, data from other states indicate that the problem is not limited to Florida or to general surgeons. Surely, the premiums cited indicate that the problem is real, but, just as surely, the variation in premiums indicates that the problem does not have a simple explanation.

Indeed, the GAO concluded that multiple factors contributed to the recent rapid increases: (1) "Since 1998 insurers' losses on medical malpractice claims have increased rapidly in some states." (2) "From 1998 through 2001 medical malpractice insurers experienced decreases in their investment income as interest rates fell on the bonds that generally make up around 80 percent of these insurers' investment portfolios." (3) "During the 1990s insurers competed vigorously for medical malpractice business, and several factors, including high investment returns, permitted them to offer prices [in pursuit of a larger "market share"] that in hindsight, for some insurers, did not completely cover their ultimate losses on that business. As a result of this, some companies became insolvent or voluntarily left the market, reducing the downward competitive pressure on premium rates." (4) "Beginning in 2001 reinsurance rates for medical malpractice insurers also increased more rapidly than they had in the past, raising insurers' overall costs."[28] In summary, the GAO explanation for premium increases rests heavily on the behavior of insurance companies rather than on frequency of claims and sizes of awards or settlements.

There is a growing literature on the various issues surrounding unintentional medical injuries, medical malpractice, litigation awards and settlements, and malpractice premiums.[29] In reading that literature it is important to recognize that, like politics, "all medical care is local." The physician who has to deal with a large malpractice insurance premium in his or her state and specialty is not made more comfortable by the knowledge that the premium would be much less in an adjoining state. This helps explain the intensity of feeling that physicians often have. Since insurance is primarily regulated by the various states and not by the federal government, and since a number of states have legislated what they (and the AMA) consider adequate responses to the problems they confront, the GAO report concluded by telling Congress that it was "not recommending executive action." However, it continued, "to further the understanding of conditions in current and future malpractice markets, Congress may wish to consider encouraging the National Association of Insurance Commissioners and state insurance regulators to identify and collect additional, mutually beneficial data necessary for evaluating the medical malpractice market." This call for research (and doing so with words that do not suggest a sense of urgency) rather than for "executive action" certainly suggests that as recently as 2003 the GAO did not view the malpractice situation as one of crisis.

We believe that the difference between the GAO and the AMA and physician perceptions stems from two factors: (1) the "crisis" has become more widespread (in the eighteen months from January 2003 to June 2004 eight states were added to the AMA's earlier crisis list of twelve);[30] (2) the GAO was addressing its report to the Congress and suggesting what it saw as appropriate federal action in an insurance arena that traditionally has "belonged" to the states. Thus it reflected a national perspective rather than state conditions.

Physician communication as well as interpersonal skills helps determine whether a patient will file a claim. Physicians who feel victimized by the existing malpractice system may feel that the suggestion that the fault lies with their communicative skills is simply another case of "blaming the victim" and may react negatively to the implied suggestion that it is important to develop and strengthen those skills. They might respond instead that the problem should not be attributed to some deficiency on their part but to the external environment that inhibits communication. First, communication and the establishment of interpersonal relations take time and, as we have discussed, physicians already feel pressured to accomplish more in fewer hours.[31] Second, claims and suits often involve a physician who is a "stranger," but that is the nature of modern medicine. Patients are treated by specialists and subspecialists, and the relationship with such doctors often involves infrequent intersections over a short time span and is likely to be different from one's relationships with a personal or primary care physician.[32] Third, the very threat of potential litigation inhibits the communication that, were it present, might alter the decision to sue. Thus communication can make a difference, but not inevitably. If the suit does go forward, the earlier communication might give the plaintiff an advantage.

It should be clear that the medical malpractice problem and the issue of premium increases are not matters to be examined as if they solely concerned a string of individual cases. One's focus must turn to a more general set of issues. The existing approach to malpractice claims has numerous deficiencies: (1) Small, but real, claims are not litigated because potential claimants, though "harmed," may be unaware of the possibility of filing a claim or be unwilling to do so, and because, given the potential award and the probability of a successful claim, attorneys who operate on the basis of contingency fees and bear the economic costs of litigation may (quite appropriately) choose not to invest the time to pursue the matter. Thus there is little, if any, compensation for a significant proportion of errors.[33] That this is not surprising does not make it less disturbing. (2) Most claims and most litigation do not result in payments to the patient, but unsuccessful claims and litigation add to the costs of the system. The fact that there are relatively few payouts does not mean that those claims were frivolous, but it does suggest there is a high overhead cost that might well be reduced by additional or alternative mechanisms to resolve disputes. (3) There is little evidence that the existing approach (as it applies to claims against physicians) has a deterrent effect; it may, in fact, be counterproductive. Evidence suggests that a significant proportion of medical errors are system rather than individual errors. If so, the inhibitions to effective communication serve to reduce the probability that system errors will be uncovered and dealt with to the benefit of future patients.

The costs of the various legal steps involved in a malpractice suit are substantial, and this is reflected in the insurance premiums. Given the variable costs of discovery and litigation and the low probability of a judgment against the defendant, one can understand the reasons that attorneys do not believe their fees are excessive; they must consider the expenses they incur in the totality of cases in which they are involved. At the same time one can understand the irritation that physicians and others often express about attorneys who, in their judgment, bring suits that are not justified (presumably, the percentage of cases that the defendant wins are evidence of that), and who then use their "failure" rate to justify very large awards in the suits in which they are successful and even rely on the juries to inflate awards because jurors know that only a portion of the award will reach the plaintiff.

Given this range of perceptions, it is not hard to conclude that procedures now in place do not serve patients or physicians well. The existing system cries for change and the validity of that need does not rest on whether a particular statistic about this or that percentage of cases does or does not really involve negligence, whether a particular datum is "correct," or how much of the explanation for premium increases can be attributed to the size of awards rather than to other considerations. Theoretical arguments can be adduced to show that we have a system that will not move us toward desired goals of equity in compensating victims of negligence, of furthering safe practices (by individuals, institutions, and systems), and of deterring unsafe ones. We also conclude that the existing system of determining premiums fails to stimulate the profession to take appropriate action to monitor its own behavior and deal with those few physicians whose performance is consistently poor.

There have been numerous proposals for fundamental reform of the tort system in medical malpractice both at the federal level and within the individual states. It may be overly optimistic to believe that such reform will be embraced in the near future (especially in a politically polarized environment) and that out of it would come a system that will deal in an equitable manner with the haphazardness of compensation for injured patients, contribute to an increase in patient safety, and reduce the costs of the malpractice system. Nevertheless, given the increase in premiums in some states and for some specialties and the impact of such changes on the availability of care, there is a need to institute corrections (even if incomplete and not comprehensive) that address these issues without delay. Not by accident a large number of initiatives have been suggested and discussed. While we are not prepared to endorse any particular set of approaches, one thing does seem clear. The problems of rising malpractice premiums and the suggestions of "crisis" are recurring ones. That does not mean that they are less pressing or that they can be dismissed in the hope that they will, as has occurred in the past, disappear. Rather, it means that though each unintentional injury and the factors contributing to it may differ, there are basic structural problems in the design of the malpractice system. A number of these structural issues require government intervention and an increase in government regulation (though it should be clear that self-regulation by the legal and the medical professions would lessen the need for some government oversight).

In bringing reform to a malpractice arena that is overlaid with emotion, it is especially necessary that changes be made on the basis of information and careful analysis rather than on the basis of anecdotes and horror stories. The existing adversarial approach to change assumes that every gain for patients and their attorneys represents a loss to physicians and insurers, and that every change that would benefit physicians would necessarily harm patients. That need not be the case.

The Decline of the American Medical Association

The absence of national medical leadership that would offer programs and policies to deal with the growth and complexity of medical care in the last third of the twentieth century added to the frustration of many physicians. The umbrella organization for all physicians was the American Medical Association, which came to be perceived by the outside world as offering knee-jerk opposition to almost any proposed innovation in the delivery and financing of medical care. Its doctrinaire opposition to virtually all governmentally sponsored programs put it at odds with elected representatives of both parties. Since it seldom proposed meaningful alternative solutions—as did the leadership of a number of specialty societies—it appeared to behave as if it either did not recognize the problems that beset medicine or preferred the status quo. Significantly, the AMA provided little evidence that it understood or was sensitive to the expressed needs of the general public. This appeared especially to be the case during the period in which Congress passed the bumper crop of health legislation in 1965. Inevitably, the organization's behavior during the debate on the two major initiatives, Medicare and Medicaid, led it to lose credibility among, or to be viewed as irrelevant by, policy makers in both the public and private sectors.[34]

Why the AMA did not emerge as a counterforce during the 1980s and 1990s to the power that had come to reside in the third-party payers (largely the insurance industry) is a matter of speculation. Most likely it resulted from the political conservatism that dominated among the AMA leaders. They believed the "market" would solve the emerging problems. This misjudgment was compounded by their intransigence in viewing government as "the enemy." As a consequence, though practitioners were subject to ever more regulation and harassment from entrepreneurs in the private sector who sought to generate ever larger profits for investors, the leaders of organized medicine generally remained passive. Their behavior continued to encourage physicians (and patients) to blame Medicare rather than private insurers for the increase in paperwork, the need for prior approvals, and for restrictions on clinical freedom. Regrettably, the leadership of the organization also committed other blunders. Perhaps most prominent was the "Sunbeam" case, in which in 1997 the AMA agreed to endorse Sunbeam's "Health at Home" products in return for a percentage of sale income. The AMA canceled the arrangement after charges of conflict of interest culminated in severe criticism and backlash. After Sunbeam brought suit for breach of contract, the matter was settled for $9.9 million.[35] A second public relations and image fiasco occurred in 1999 when the AMA dismissed George Lundberg, the editor of the *Journal of the American Medical Association* (who had served in that capacity for seventeen years), because of his decision to publish an article that the AMA Board of Trustees felt was inappropriate (even if scientifically correct). The event was widely viewed as an example of political interference with editorial autonomy.[36]

The growing lack of confidence in the AMA among physicians was one of the factors that led to a decline in membership. In 1972 seventy-five percent of all physicians were members of the AMA; thirty years later this was true of only twenty-nine percent. As a consequence of this precipitous decline, in 2003 the organization's Board of Trustees commissioned a study to explore the feasibility of the AMA's becoming a federation of the existing specialty organizations (which, in contrast with the AMA, had expanded over the same time period). Useful as such a change might have been for the Association, it was difficult to discern why the members of these specialty organizations would desire to cast their lot with the AMA, an organization that many of them had elected not to join. In any event, the proposed federation was rejected by the House of Delegates of the AMA. Had it occurred, it might have proven beneficial to American medicine and to the general public. With a new organizational structure and with new leadership (especially if drawn from the specialty societies, which, in a number of cases, had proven far more open on issues of health care access and insurance than had the AMA), there would have been the potential for the Association to become more responsive to the needs of its own physician membership and, importantly, to the needs of the broader community.

The failure of leadership at the American Medical Association should not obscure the fact that many physicians who were very busy taking care of patients, shouldering more and more time-consuming administrative burdens, and maintaining their skills in the face of an explosion in the knowledge base, were concerned about the organizational and financial issues troubling American medicine. In the late 1980s a number of physicians, generally younger ones, organized Physicians for a National Health Program (PNHP), which advocated universal insurance via a single payer health plan.[37] Other physicians have formed statewide organizations to deal with access issues in their localities. Still others have found outlets for their social concerns through participation in such organizations as the International Physicians to Prevent Nuclear War, which was awarded the Nobel Peace Prize in 1985. Its United States arm, Physicians for Social Responsibility, serves as an advocate for various public health policies, many of them related to violence and to environmental issues.

In the national interest, as well as in its own self-interest, the medical profession needs to find an organizational format that reflects the pluralism of its membership. Without this, it will continue on a course of diffuseness and fragmentation in which it exerts little influence on the shaping of health policy. There is an array of issues that American medicine could and should debate and on which it should present its views: the financing of health services for the uninsured,[38] the simplification of both private and public administrative procedures by third-party payers, the recognition of the importance of preventive services, and the adequate funding of the public health infrastructure. A failure to participate in debates over these and other issues and a continuation of its posture of looking toward the past instead of toward the future will, unfortunately, further marginalize most American physicians. As a consequence the national debates will be less informed, and both physicians and the public will be the losers.

The Continuing Search for New Knowledge

During the twentieth century medical care and public health were transformed by new technologies resulting from advances in biomedical research. The support for much of this research came from public sources, especially the National Institutes of Health. Universities, research institutions, scientists, citizens' groups, and congressional action all reflected a widespread interest in this endeavor and a national consensus that biomedical research was a social good. There was little discussion of how much is enough, although occasional concerns were expressed about the capacity to use all the funds effectively.[39]

Though some critics regard the NIH governance process as ponderous and relatively inflexible,[40] its scientific enterprise has proven to be remarkably creative. Perhaps the organization's eclectic approach to science and pragmatic management explains how it has both maintained stability while fostering creativity. It may well be that the public involvement in the direction of the NIH has been its major source of strength. It, of course, is true that large organizations, and NIH is a large organization, often find it difficult to be entirely transparent, and in recent years (in part as the result of the increasingly close interrelationships between the public and the private research sectors) NIH has had to face its own conflict-of-interest issues.[41] These problems are deeply troubling both because of their substance and because of their symbolic value since NIH has long been viewed as an organization driven only by scientific criteria of the highest order. While NIH has adopted new and explicit standards to govern future behavior, the recent revelations argue strongly that an even more open process, though cumbersome, would serve as an important source of protection.

As a consequence of the considerable public and, more recently, private investment in research, medical practitioners have moved from an earlier period when, as in the first half of the twentieth century, few specific therapies were available to a period in which innovative and potent diagnostic and therapeutic technologies are burgeoning. Accessing this knowledge has been facilitated by the revolution in telecommunications, which makes it possible for a practitioner to readily retrieve the current literature and protocols for patient management. A logical consequence of the new scientific knowledge has been the expansion of the medical-industrial sector whose commitments to "development" have been important in translating laboratory findings into available products. In a reciprocal manner the sector has contributed to the new knowledge and, of course, to the various therapies that flowed from it. Instrument makers and pharmaceutical companies have benefited from the basic research sponsored by the NIH and have engaged in vigorous product development.

As we have already discussed, the potential profitability of research findings and their "translation" have not been lost on biomedical scientists in the academic world. As a result conflicts of interest have increased both in frequency and significance. Regrettably, the task of reducing these conflicts and of policing the system is difficult given the large number of universities, hospitals, and research institutions. The potential monetary gains to individual faculty members, as well as the number of dollars involved, are great, and faculty members, bench researchers, and clinical investigators are quite mobile. Strict rules in one university may lead the investigator to pack his or her bags and move on to an institution with looser ones. Nevertheless, because there is so much at stake, every effort must be made to develop collective guidelines that all adhere to, to set high standards even at some cost, and to do a much better job than has been done in the past of explaining the bases for those standards to new entrants into the profession. Whereas in the past, medical school and hospital administrators may have believed faculty members and clinical staff subscribed to a set of common and widely held values, they can no longer make that assumption. In a world in which medicine is often viewed as just one more "product," one in which commerce and commercialism seem to have invaded every sphere of our economic, political, and social life, traditional values can no longer be taken for granted.

University administrators realize that the close ties between the academy and the private medical-industrial sector as well as the involvements of faculty members in commercial ventures are here to stay, in part because, though troubling, they are beneficial to the scientific endeavor. These academic leaders must be prepared to develop and offer their own incentives that may help reduce the temptations to ignore conflicts of interest in order to maximize income, prestige, and stock options. If they fail, the university will have failed its students and the greater society. Once students cannot partake in the interplay of ideas because faculty members cannot share "trade secrets," the basic trust and openness of the university will be no more.

Society will be the loser since the privileges it has granted to institutions of higher learning and to the members of such institutions have been conferred on the assumption that in return the community of scholars will produce things of value (books, research, and ideas) to be shared by all. Indeed, the institution of academic freedom was designed to protect scholars so that they could produce such contributions as they saw fit and be uncontrolled by the heavy hands even of donors and benefactors. Academic freedom was bestowed not only because it was important to the academicians who received it, but because it was important to the society that granted it. It enabled the academician to be the social critic and the purveyor of ideas, and the society at large was wise enough to know it would be the beneficiary. Thus the battle in and around the (inevitable) conflicts of interest that arise is a battle for the soul of the institutions in which future physicians are trained, future therapies are discovered, and today's patients are treated.[42] It is a battle we dare not lose.

Toward a Comprehensive Delivery System: Bringing Order out of Chaos

Health care cannot be delivered without resources. Resources cannot function in an effective and efficient manner without organization and structure. While it sometimes is tempting to imagine that all that stands between today's dysfunctional health care system and one that we could all boast about and be pleased with is the enactment and implementation of a universal health insurance program, that is not the case. Important as the development of an effective universal program that removed the economic barriers that many face when they seek medical care would be, it would still prove insufficient. The removal of financial barriers would not assure that the health care system would be transformed into a model of efficiency, one that would deliver comprehensive services of high quality that met the needs of the population while not wasting resources. Other changes would be required to bring order out of the chaos that now characterizes much of the American health care system.

Some of the legislative changes that we advocate will appear familiar to those who have followed developments in the health care system over the last forty years. As already discussed, a number of these measures were partially or temporarily implemented at earlier times. The fact that they were tried and either did not work as well as had been anticipated or were repealed or not renewed (sometimes in spite of the fact that they did work) should not lead us to reject them on the grounds of "been there, done that." Sometimes measures come at an inappropriate time, sometimes they need refinement. Sometimes they fail or are rejected for reasons that have little to do with their efficacy.

Sometimes those that work, but haltingly and with difficulty, can be fine-tuned to be more effective.

The various recommendations in the report of the Carnegie Commission of 1970, recommendations that urged planning for and adoption of a regional approach to the distribution of health services with academic health centers as the hubs, came to naught. Although this and similar reports still embody numerous valid and useful proposals, they have not been implemented in any systematic way. We are convinced that the nation has learned much since the Carnegie Commission report, and that one of the things it has learned is the importance of rationalizing existing health resources based upon comprehensive regionalization. Community-based primary care services need to be linked with community hospitals, diagnostic clinics, and medical center specialized services. Those linkages (including linkages between diagnostic clinics and community hospitals with medical centers) must include referral of discharged as well as of sick patients.[43] Because of the rapid advances in research, the expansion of specialized services has been relatively greater in recent years and has amplified the necessity for regionalization and regional planning even beyond what it was at the time of the Carnegie report. The question is not whether the need is even clearer. The question is whether that knowledge has made action more acceptable and more likely.

Over time and in a pragmatic fashion, the United States has evolved a network of academic health science centers, which in addition to meeting their responsibilities for the education and training of health professionals and the delivery of clinical care, are the locus of much of the nation's biomedical research activity.[44] As a consequence these vital hubs of our system bear intertwined responsibilities in patient care, education and training, and basic and clinical research.

Because many of these academic health centers are geographically dispersed, a process is needed to assure an appropriate inflow of patients. This concern is obvious in the case of medical centers (often associated with state universities) that are sparsely located in areas with relatively small populations. It is also true, however, in large urban areas that may offer any number of medical centers. While it has been argued that competition between such centers has improved the quality of care and lowered costs, we do not believe that experience bears this out. Excess capacity is generated as each urban center attempts to get a larger market share and as the total supply of diagnostic equipment, hospital beds, and therapeutic resources grows beyond that needed to serve the total population. This is wasteful and leads to increases in expenditures.[45]

Furthermore, without a mechanism to coordinate the flow of patients and to match facilities and resources to population and demographic needs, some centers might have too low a volume of patients to meet their teaching needs and, even more important, too few to be able to perform highly specialized services at an appropriate level of quality. The fact that some states have tried to improve the quality of care by monitoring outcomes and eliminating services that have poor volume and meager records of outcomes again suggests an important role for planning and for cooperation between and among the various units of the American health care system.

Since many academic health centers conduct regional programs, it would seem appropriate to modulate the allocation of resources and the flow of patients through the regional commissions we have already referred to in discussing educational assistance and that will be discussed more fully in presenting our ideas on the ways to achieve universal insurance. While there inevitably will be a measure of anxiety about a strong regulatory process and the implied "politicization," public representation and input would help assure that these regional commissions carry on their activities in a transparent fashion, act in the public's interest, and are held accountable. In a sense this would cast medical care's research and development functions (as well as the provision of health care) in a public utility framework. Both the national commission and regional subcommissions would have the responsibility for assuring equity without operating any aspect of the system.

Our suggestions clearly call for more planning and for an infrastructure that would make effective planning possible. We believe that, as in education, fire and police protection, highways, and other public goods, it is contradictory to acknowledge, on the one hand, that services should be provided on a universal basis, yet maintain on the other that their provision need not be planned and instead can be left to untrammeled market forces. If, for example, government states that every child should have an adequate education, it is government's responsibility to assure that the resources that would make that education possible are in place. That responsibility is not always met, but the problem is addressed not by denying government's responsibility, but by developing the political will to meet it. Furthermore, since the nation has multiple needs, it also is government's responsibility to assure that resources are not wasted and that we do not spend more than is required to achieve the educational (or other) goals that society has set.

These same criteria hold for health care. Regrettably, there is no political consensus (in an operational rather than a rhetorical sense) that health care is a right. If, however, as a society we do subscribe to the view that health care is a right, we cannot leave it to the market to enable or enforce it. To confer a right is to accept a responsibility to make it operative. We strongly believe that conscientious planning is preferable to the entrepreneurial expansions (including many mergers and acquisitions) that have characterized our recent past.

Beyond the Hubs

The settings in which health care is delivered have become more diverse and complex over the past several decades. Some fifty years ago Dr. Fein studied the factors that influenced the location decisions of general practitioners in North Carolina. The same physicians were interviewed twenty-five years later and asked to describe their practice and how things had worked out. It was startling to note that in the original interviews there was little mention of the hospital as an institution whose presence or quality had entered into the location decision. These physicians did not expect the hospital to be an important locus of their activity. This had changed by the time of the set of second interviews. These revealed that the hospital had become a critical part of the physicians' professional lives. Though still general practitioners, their offices were close to the hospital, and they spent a considerable proportion of their time inside its walls and, as a consequence, with other physicians.[46] Although it is still possible to find communities that are served by solo practitioners or small partnerships, most physicians practice in some group setting (such as an HMO) or as part of a network of physicians (such as preferred provider organizations). Still others practice in publicly funded community health centers, health department clinics, community hospital outpatient clinics, or in programs of the Department of Veterans Affairs. In short, physicians seldom practice alone.

The model for medical care that has evolved is one in which the patient has a continuing relationship with a community-based primary care physician. These physicians are regarded as generalists and come from a variety of "primary care specialties" such as pediatrics, internal medicine, and obstetrics in addition to family practice. These generalists have relationships to various specialists (cardiologists, general surgeons, urologists, neurologists, dermatologists, and so forth) who are also based in the community, and who can be distinguished from the subspecialist consultants who are found in academic health centers. The large and increasing number of specialists and subspecialists reflects the greater knowledge base available for modern medical care. Yet this augmentation means that inevitably, and appropriately, patients intersect with any number of physicians. If hospitalized in an academic medical center, the patient may quite legitimately be confused as to whether the primary care physician (that is, the patient's "regular" physician) or the academic consultant is the critical decision maker. The busy primary care physician, therefore, has a new and most important role: to integrate the services provided by the several specialists while acting as the point of reference for the patient.

This arrangement sounds logical and, though involving many relationships, perhaps quite simple. Yet it will come as no surprise to discover that the primary care physician does not find it simple to serve as the reference point and coordinator. The fact that patients need a physician coordinator does not translate into a clear system response. There is an important missing link: insurers do not pay for "coordinating" services. HMOs, concerned about restraining premium growth and meeting the "competition," call for more patients per hour, shorter visits, and less conversation—policies that are at variance with the need to facilitate the patient's negotiating the necessary specialized services and consultations.

In part as a response to the willingness and ability of some patients to pay on their own for such services, in part out of physician frustration at not having the time or encouragement to practice the kind of medicine (at the more leisurely pace) that many of them desire and believe is called for (without risking loss of income), some physicians are providing what has come to be termed "concierge medicine." Under this arrangement the patient is required to "sign up" with the physician and pay a flat annual fee (usually some thousands of dollars) to the physician or the physician group. This fee is not tied to specific encounters or service; rather, it is more like a club membership. The physician receives that flat sum as well as insurance or other payments that would be billed for specific interventions. In return for the already paid-for ticket of admission, the physician agrees to provide the most precious commodity: time. He or she is able to do so because the physician's practice is limited to a (relatively) small number of patients. Yet the physician's income is not reduced (indeed, may be increased) because of the "membership" fee.[47]

When successful, that is, when the physician is able to sign up the requisite number of patients, the various parties (patients and physicians) presumably have what they seek: an opportunity to have interactions of the kind that they imagine took place in the "good old days" without the economic pressures that they forget existed even then. It should be clear, however, that this arrangement does not provide a generalizable answer to the problem involved in patient-physician interactions, the issues raised by specialization and subspecialization, and the behaviors of reimbursing agencies. Because the entrance fee has to be substantial (in order to permit the physician to have a much lower patient load), this model can be available only to a limited affluent segment of the population. That, of course, is why it has been labeled "concierge medicine." Furthermore, if the model were to spread and become commonplace, those persons in the general community who could not or did not opt for this approach would be left with fewer physicians to serve their needs. The arithmetic is clear: if there are more physicians for the most affluent members of the community, there will be fewer physicians for the rest of the population. Thus concierge medicine does not represent another "patch" on the system; rather, if it were to grow significantly, it would represent a threat to the viability of the existing system and a threat as well to the goal of a more equitable delivery system. Its spread is not a solution; instead it is a symptom of a deep-seated problem.

Yet the need for greater patient/physician interaction remains. As a consequence over the past several decades there has been considerable exploration of the utility of training nonphysician professionals to take over some of the physician's responsibilities for primary care, with a concomitant growth in programs for nurse-practitioners and physician assistants. State licensure standards have developed to sanction such professionals to provide medical care, generally in settings under the supervision of physicians. Similarly, there have been substantial increases in the number of licensed clinical psychologists and social workers. Once again we are reminded of the utility of the prepaid group practice model in which these kinds of personnel can more readily be utilized, supervised, and integrated. There is little question that the PGP approach makes it possible to rationalize the health care tasks that various types of personnel can perform, thereby providing more services with the given resources and improving the effectiveness and output of physicians, the scarcest resource.

In recent years HMOs have acquired a bad name, one that never attached to prepaid group practices over all the decades in which they existed. Reputation aside, the fact is that many HMOs can provide efficient care of high quality and utilize fewer resources in doing so. The tragedy is that the bad name was acquired not because of the inherent characteristics of health maintenance organizations, but because, in the face of employer desire to control premium growth and investor desire to maximize rates of return, a number of HMOs were prepared to deny service and emphasize profits to the detriment of patients and the values of medicine. Furthermore, facing the same employer imperatives and competitive pressure from for-profits, some not-for-profit HMOs were forced to compromise their standards and their reputations. The consequences are distressing because there is a danger that the HMO model has fallen into disfavor and may be discarded for the wrong reasons, that is, in spite of the fact that it is an effective way to organize part of the medical care delivery system.

Many HMOs are appendages of insurance companies and view themselves as organizations that manage the flow of dollars rather than as organizations that manage the delivery of care; that being the case, it is difficult to be optimistic about prospects for a return to the values that once impelled non-profit prepaid group practice. For that to occur would require pressure from multiple sources: (1) subscribers who are paying an increasing share of the premium and face higher levels of cost-sharing deductibles, co-pays, and co-insurance; (2) employers who want to gain a competitive edge that is related to the quality of care their employees receive; and (3) physicians who entered medicine with a sense of idealism about service and who are distressed at the commercialization of their chosen profession. It will also require involvement by government at all levels, for it is government that represents the people and, importantly, is paying for the care of millions of Medicare beneficiaries and Medicaid recipients, and (often at the local and state level) for millions of uninsured. It is clear that with multiple sources of health care funding, in which no single payer has great leverage, government cannot stand on the sidelines and, unwilling to exert its power and potential leadership, wait for some nonexistent catalyst to appear and mobilize that diverse constituency.

Government has many roles to play in helping to plan and organize an efficient and comprehensive delivery system, yet that system would be for naught if the public were unable to access the services the system could provide. We now turn to the role that government can play in assuring that all Americans have access and the necessary financial protection to help meet the high and rising costs of care.

8 | Increasing Equity: Achieving Universal Health Insurance

The most recent major effort to enact a comprehensive universal insurance program was the Clinton plan of 1993. As discussed earlier, while many factors contributed to its failure of adoption, especially significant was the growth and concomitant power of the insurance industry and of its lobbying capacities. The industry exploited the general ambivalence about government's ability to manage large-scale programs (perhaps captured most cynically in the bumper sticker, "If You Like the Post Office You'll Love National Health Insurance"). Earlier positive attitudes toward government's capacities, as reflected in public approval of the Manhattan Project and the mission to land a person on the moon, had given way among many Americans to the conviction that "nothing works." Furthermore, the insurance industry also succeeded in purveying the notion that, given free reign and not bound by "onerous" regulations, the private sector could and would solve major social policy problems. This, of course, was before 2002–2003, when the public became aware of the many examples of mismanagement and corruption in industry (including the health care industry) and on Wall Street.

With the failure to enact the Clinton program (it did not reach the floor of either chamber of Congress), with the threat of "big government" removed—indeed, in his 1996 State of the Union address President Clinton took pride in proclaiming that "the era of big government is over"—the nation chose (or was forced) to rely on free-market competition as the solution to the various health issues the United States faced: the problems of the uninsured, the maldistribution of resources, and the rapidly escalating health care expenditures. To the nation's regret, the free market failed to provide the needed remedies. The "business" of the new health entrepreneurs was not that of solving social problems, but of making money. It became apparent that, in spite of its presumed ideological virtue, reliance on competition did little to control the continuing escalation of expenditures, redistribute resources, or expand insurance coverage. The nation learned that the new health economy could not resolve the various inequities within the health care system.

None of this should have come as a surprise. The market is not a redistributive device, and many of the health problems required some, and in a number of cases much, redistribution. The market responds to disparities in income and allocates resources to meet market demand (the exercise of which requires income) rather than to meet needs (a concept with which economists, as economists, have difficulty). Yet health issues are about "need," not about the economic concept of "demand." The latter can be measured; the former is a matter of opinion. Nevertheless, that does not make "need" any less real. Although Americans seemed to agree that health care was a "right," and did not embrace the counter-formulation that health care is a "privilege," the laissez-faire market still repeated, "follow the money."[1]

Furthermore, the delivery of health care services constituted a special market that did not meet the various criteria usually cited by economists for a fully competitive market. Resources could not be moved freely. New firms did not have the ease of entry that, through competition, would help constrain prices and profits. The symmetry between buyer and seller was absent since the patient (buyer) had much less knowledge than the physician (seller). Indeed, as already discussed, the real buyer often was not the consumer/patient but the employer; the managed care entity, not the physician/hospital, was the seller. In addition, there had to be many sellers, no single one large or powerful enough to influence market supply significantly, as well as many purchasers, no single one large or powerful enough to influence demand significantly. True, in the nation overall and in the various states individually there were many hospitals, many HMOs, and many insurers, all together presumably making for competition. Nevertheless, the health care market that most of us faced and in which most health care was produced and delivered was in fact a local market. Many local markets had a very limited number of health institutions and of organized delivery systems. Thus those who sought and received medical care in their localities (and that, of course, meant most of us most of the time) did not necessarily face conditions that rendered a competitive market possible.

Though the market failed to provide "the" answer to the problems the nation faced in health care delivery, the rejection of the Clinton program did not inspire any renewed attempts to enact comprehensive legislation. The political landscape did not encourage the kind of sustained, patient effort that characterized the years that it took to enact Medicare. In the face of a divided Congress, amid the political distraction created by impeachment, and without any political consensus on the criteria that major change should embody, public policy turned to incrementalism. With no solutions forthcoming from market forces, band-aids and patches were applied to perceived problems. Each patch was at best helpful, but none was integrated into a coherent comprehensive plan. Employers who provided health insurance for their employees shopped for lower-cost plans that often disrupted the continuity of medical care of their employees. Insurers attempted to deal with rising costs and premiums by establishing or expanding various co-payments and/or deductibles. Inevitably, these cost-sharing devices, designed to make the patient more cost-conscious and therefore reduce utilization, aggravated the complexity of accessing the system for both patients and professionals.

Legislatively, though various incremental measures have been enacted in the decade since the Clinton program was put forward, it has been forty years since the last two major health initiatives, Medicare and Medicaid, were passed by Congress in 1965.[2] It is useful to remember that was a time of great social ferment, particularly as a consequence of the civil rights revolution and the War on Poverty, and there was political will for bold social action. Since then there has been little political appetite for comprehensive solutions, as is evident in the failure of the Nixon, Carter, and Clinton proposals. Instead, piecemeal efforts prevail, such as legislation to create HMOs, improve "portability" of health insurance between jobs, and, more recently, offer better provisions for health insurance for children through the states (the

State Children's Health Insurance Program). As a consequence of the failure to enact comprehensive legislation, we are left with an arrangement in which power is dispersed among health professionals, corporate entities representing hospitals and insurance industries, pharmaceutical and medical device manufacturers, and, of course, a variety of governmental agencies. Reasonable people debate whether we in effect have a health care "system" or "nonsystem."

Who Are the Uninsured and What Care Do They Receive?

The most significant problem, that of providing health insurance (and through health insurance, greater access to health services) for 45 million uninsured persons, tragically continues to be neglected. Though the number of "uninsured" is critical, it is subject to wavering definition—specifically, how long does an individual need to be without insurance before he or she is counted. Whatever the definition, the resulting number is large and has increased (and continues to increase) in recent years as a consequence of declining employment in manufacturing industries that typically provide health insurance benefits, the creation of new jobs in service industries that do not offer health insurance, and employer health insurance cutbacks in the face of rising premiums and a weakened labor movement.

Readers may have their own impressions (and misimpressions) about the characteristics of the uninsured population. Dr. Fein recalls being interviewed by a reporter for one of the national weekly news magazines. With some exasperation the interviewer stated that he did not believe what he had heard about the uninsured—all of his friends had insurance, and he wasn't certain that the uninsured really existed. It was suggested that he cross the street and interview the help at the pizza parlor, or at the diner, or the hamburger joint, or the shoe repair shop, and inquire about their health insurance coverage. The reporter came back shaken. It was his first encounter with that part of the "real world." He was especially troubled about the shoe repairman, who was a new father of only a few weeks' duration and had confided that he hoped his child would stay healthy since he had no insurance or savings. While it is true that statistics about the uninsured are somewhat aseptic and not especially gripping ("statistics are people with the tears wiped dry"),[3] the data are illuminating.

In 2003 there were 45 million Americans (up from 43.6 million in 2002), including 8.4 million children under age eighteen, without insurance.[4] Six out of ten of the uninsured between ages eighteen and sixty-five were full-year, full-time workers. Large firms are more likely to offer coverage to their employees than is the case for smaller firms. Nevertheless, a quarter of the uninsured worked, though not necessarily full-time, for firms (or were dependants of individuals who worked for firms) with over 500 employees. It is a myth that working for a large firm means one inevitably will be covered. Similarly, it is a myth that most of the uninsured are members of a minority group. It is true that almost one-third of Hispanics (and 70 percent of working-age Hispanic immigrants who have been in the United States less than five years) were uninsured. And while that was the case for one in five blacks, Asians, and Pacific Islanders, it was so for "only" one in ten non-Hispanic whites. Nevertheless, almost three-quarters of the total of uninsured persons were non-Hispanic whites.[5] Importantly, the phenomenon of the large number of uninsured is found in a nation whose per capita expenditures for health care and whose health care expenditures as a percentage of its Gross Domestic Product are considerably higher than in any other industrialized nation. On the one hand, we are the only country without universal entitlement to health care services and thus have a large number of uninsured. On the other, we spend far more on health care, both per capita and as a percentage of GDP, than does any other country.

One should not infer, however, that the uninsured do not receive any health services; rather, they receive fewer services than the insured population does, and much of that care takes place in emergency rooms and through many other ad hoc arrangements. It is estimated that in 2004 per capita medical spending for individuals insured for the full year was 180 percent higher than for persons uninsured for the full year, and 120 percent higher than for those uninsured for part of the year.[6] The uninsured, it is reported, "receive less preventive care, are diagnosed at more advanced disease states, and, once diagnosed, tend to receive less therapeutic care, and have higher mortality rates."[7] Because care for the uninsured is fragmented, incomplete, and often postponed until absolutely necessary, many low-income uninsured enter the hospital sicker than the insured and, as a consequence, stay longer, thereby in many instances adding more to costs than would have been the case had they been treated earlier.

Indeed, the expenditures on behalf of the uninsured are already so large that it is estimated that the new or additional costs that would have to be incurred to provide the uninsured with comprehensive insurance would increase the $2 trillion total national health spending by less than 3 percent ($48 billion).[8] At present the costs of uncompensated care—services delivered but not paid for by the patient or insurer (totaling some $40.7 billion, with hospital care accounting for 60 percent)—are met in various ways. One example is cost-shifting, a process by which costs incurred (but not met) are built into charges that are passed on through insurance companies to all other payers, that is, to individual subscribers and to employers who contribute to health insurance and, by reduction in wages, to their employees. Since it is reasonable to assume that providing preventive services and earlier interventions will in the long run be cost-saving, public economic interests, as well as humane considerations, argue that collectively we would all benefit if everyone had health insurance that provided for regular, comprehensive health care.

Jack Hadley and John Holahan cite a variety of studies to document the impact of not having insurance:[9] (1) "A conservative estimate based on the full range of studies is that a reduction of mortality of 5–15% could be expected if the uninsured were to gain continuous health coverage."[10] (2) "The number of excess deaths among uninsured adults age 25–64 is in the range of 18,000 per year."[11] (3) "The annual economic value of foregone health among the 40 million uninsured in 2000 has been estimated to be between $65 and $130 billion in that year."[12] Even the lower bound of the estimate ($69 billion in 2004 dollars) is considerably over the sum of $48 billion required to provide coverage to all the uninsured. It is clear that America's failure to enact universal insurance is not one of economics but of politics. We can "afford" it, but we choose other priorities (including lower taxes). We have the dollars—what we lack is the political will.

How We Got Here

The history of the financing of health services in the United States illustrates that "timing is everything" and why it has been difficult to achieve universal enrollment. In general, other industrialized nations adopted their universal financing programs (usually beginning with coverage for hospitalization expenses) before private sector insurance coverage expanded. Thus, when these nations opted for public or public-private financing of health care (under social insurance or, in any case, with a major role for the public authority), it was not necessary to dismantle the private insurance industry. Conversely, the United States was a latecomer to the concept of health insurance in general and public financing in particular. America's social insurance program, Medicare, was not implemented until 1966, almost two decades after Britain created its universal National Health Service, which covered the entire population, and five years after all Canadian provinces had adopted universal hospital insurance for the entire population (by 1972 the Canadian federal government was sharing the costs of provision of physician services in all provinces, and in 1984 the federal legislature unanimously enacted the Canada Health Act, which effectively banned extra billing and user charges).

It is unnecessary to review the detailed history of the development and growth of private health insurance or of public insurance and payment programs in the United States in order to understand the choices and constraints before the nation. It is useful, however, to summarize our earlier discussion and remind ourselves of some of the critical decisions that were made during the course of that history, decisions that have deeply affected the development of the financing and organization of American health care. Often these decisions were taken to meet specific conditions then prevailing and not because in the long run they would necessarily lead to salutary developments. Nevertheless, the fact that they may have made sense only in the short term does not negate their importance (and, on occasion, negative implications) in the long term. They have shaped the health system we encounter.

1. While health insurance had existed (largely in isolated pockets with special employment and/or geographic characteristics) in the United States before 1929, the spread of modern American health insurance dates from that time. Importantly, health insurance was initially linked to employment, thus enabling the employer to assume the administrative tasks of enrollment and collection of the premiums. This established the health insurance-employment link as "the" norm.

2. Hospital insurance expanded from this early beginning and, over time, evolved into Blue Cross. The Blues (in the various states) offered service benefits (for example, so many days in hospital) rather than indemnity benefits (so many dollars for every day in hospital). Notably, they were not treated as traditional insurance companies by state regulators. Considered a community enterprise, they employed "community-rated" premiums: all purchasers paid the same premium regardless of their demographic or other characteristics. Blue Shield plans covering physician services were a later addition to the health insurance mix.

3. Health insurance spread during World War II when wages and prices were stabilized in an effort to control inflationary pressures but employers were permitted to increase their provision of health insurance and to consider those premium payments as legitimate costs of doing business. The high rate of taxation of excess profits meant that the conferral of health insurance was largely underwritten by the federal government. This helped strengthen the concept of employer contribution to health insurance as a fringe benefit.

4. In the period following the war, changes in the regulations of the National Labor Relations Board (NLRB) and in the Internal Revenue tax code provided further important incentives to the growth and expansion of private voluntary health insurance. The NLRB ruled that employers had to recognize health insurance as a legitimate bargaining issue. Furthermore, though the tax code permitted

employers to consider health insurance premium payments as a cost of operating the enterprise, these premium contributions were not considered part of employees' taxable incomes. Thus employees would receive greater benefits if employers purchased health insurance than if the employee received that amount in wages, paid taxes, and bought insurance with the remainder.

5. These changes expanded the market for health insurance and led to the entry of for-profit insurers. These new entrants were able to compete, in part, because they offered indemnity benefits, which, though they might not provide as much coverage, could be offered at lower premiums. Most significantly, they departed from the traditional "community-rated" model by substituting "experience-rated" premiums. These premiums were based on the health experience (and health care costs) of the particular insured group. Thus the healthier the group, the lower the premium. This tended to fragment health insurance and provided an incentive to "disengage" from those who were at higher risk, among whom were the sick and the aged.

6. The pressure to provide health insurance for the aged grew since most individuals age sixty-five and over had no health insurance. A universal program that covered all the aged (Medicare) was enacted in 1965, together with a program for some of the poor (Medicaid). These two programs could be considered a "natural experiment" since Medicare was federal and virtually universal (for those sixty-five and above), while Medicaid operated within each state under state rules, regulations, and standards (though meeting federal requirements and guidelines) and was limited to the poor (an ever-changing population). Medicare was governed by a social insurance philosophy that spoke of "beneficiaries"; Medicaid was governed by a welfare approach that spoke of "recipients." Regrettably, public policy has not built on the results of this experiment in determining policy.

7. The increase in medical care utilization, as a consequence of the expanding power of medicine to assist the sick and because of the spread of private and public health insurance, helped fuel an increase in both per capita costs and in the share of the GDP repre-

sented by the health sector. The growing pressure on costs, premiums, and public and private expenditures resulted in attempts to move away from traditional fee-for-service medicine in which the costs were directly related to the number and intensity of the services provided in the particular physician visit or hospital stay. This led to the development of HMOs and to the later establishment of the Diagnostic Related Group (DRG) system for hospital payment.

8. The growth in the absolute number of dollars and in the percent of the GDP accounted for by the health sector attracted the attention of for-profit entities and of venture capital. The result was an expansion of for-profit hospitals, short-term nursing homes, long-term care institutions, and HMOs. A new language was introduced into the world of medical care: physicians became providers or producers, patients became customers or consumers, medical services became profit (or loss) centers, and in the case of traditional not-for-profit community hospitals, an excess of income over expenditures was explicitly termed "profit."[13] If words affect attitudes and attitudes affect behavior, it can be argued that in adopting the language of the marketplace, the health sector first introduced and later adapted to a different value system.

9. Over several decades there have been numerous attempts to establish a universal health insurance program that would cover all of the population. Though the goal remained universality, the specific mechanisms to achieve that goal proposed by various administrations were different. The approach that has received the most attention from those Presidents who submitted proposals over the last four decades has built on the existing employment linkage by "mandating" employer coverage. That system would require that most employers provide health insurance to their employees, and would provide other mechanisms to cover those employees working for firms that were not covered by the mandate—typically, small, low-wage, and not very profitable enterprises.

This brief survey and the important events and developments it describes set the stage for our discussion of universal health insurance, the system that would provide coverage not only for the 45 million

Americans without any private or public health insurance and the millions of others who, by any reasonable standard, have inadequate insurance, but for all who (absent the universal program) might become uninsured or underinsured in the future. We may wish that the United States health financing system had evolved differently, that there had been a different history, that at various times we had taken other decisions and had gone down other paths, but that did not happen. We might also wish that various political leaders had engaged in more vigorous and more sustained battle for universal coverage, that the public had been better organized and more vocal in its support for change, and that the political system had been more responsive. Nevertheless, conjecture about what might have been does not remove the constraints generated by what is. In similar fashion, some would wish that we were more like Canadians since Canada has had a universal provincial system for decades. Wishes, however, do not make it possible to behave as if we and our Canadian neighbors share a common history, set of attitudes toward government, and culture. Undoubtedly, there is much that we can learn from the Canadian experience, but we are not "Canadian," and the opportunities we face and have faced have been molded by our experiences, not theirs.

We begin by sketching what we believe represents the most desirable approach to universal coverage. This shall serve as the "benchmark," the standard from which to compromise when compromise is necessary. That, however, is not sufficient. Realism requires that we move beyond the description of the sort of plan that, in some abstract world, we would favor on grounds of equity and efficiency. We need to describe a set of program characteristics that would meet our objective of universal coverage while at the same time respecting the constraints that we believe arise from the financing and organization of existing arrangements and from the nature of the American political system.

We believe the financing and organization of the American health care delivery system are badly flawed. The link between insurance coverage and employment has impeded the achievement of equity in coverage and access, and has had deleterious effects on labor negotiations, labor peace, and economic competition. The fact that insurance companies also deliver health care (the typical for-profit HMO arrangement) has introduced a third party whose concern is maximizing profit into the medical encounter, and has led to a weakening of the role of clinical judgment and freedom. The utilization of private insurance companies to bear risk (rather than, as in Medicare, using government as the "underwriter" for all who are in the program) has provided an incentive to fractionate the insurance pool and to exclude those with preexisting conditions, those who are more likely to need medical care, and (when we gain more knowledge) those whose genes suggest they have a higher than average risk of illness and disease. The expansion of the for-profit sector has called into question the historic and valuable trust relationship between physician and patient and has had constraining effects on the physician's exercise of appropriate clinical judgment. The reliance on market competition in allocating medical care resources has resulted in the closure of many facilities, especially those operating under public auspices. Absent sound planning (and it is absent), the closures are not determined in relation to community needs, but in relation to market tests, tests that the facilities serving the poor and the uninsured are much less likely to meet.

Resolving Basic Options

In considering the American health system, the need for and the nature of desired and possible changes, the nation will need to resolve some basic issues that will ultimately inform the detailed design of a universal insurance plan and guide its blueprint. We describe here a number of these issues.

The first deals with the issue of comprehensive as contrasted with incremental change. There are reasons to argue that the American political system is not conducive to comprehensive change. Honorable persons, including many who favor a comprehensive solution, feel that in the American system one can attain such a goal only through a series of discrete (and even small) steps, and that unwillingness to devote effort to partial solutions harms those who might be helped today. Nor does resistance to incremental change bring the comprehensive solution and the goal of universal coverage any closer.

Reasonable as that view is, there are others who argue that health care system problems cannot be solved in piecemeal fashion, if only because a fundamental attribute of any comprehensive program must be that it address the issue of cost containment. They believe that programs that expand coverage in modest ways and to one group at a time do little to remake the health care system and, therefore, are unable to address cost issues in an effective and equitable manner. This view draws on the analogy that the health care system is like a balloon: if you push it here, it pops out there. They reject the old saying that half a loaf is better than none. They suggest instead that, though half a loaf may be preferable, how does one judge whether what one is debating is half a loaf, or less, or more, and how does one determine whether accepting half a loaf raises or lowers the probability of acquiring the whole loaf?

Those voicing yet another point of view accept the notion that the American political system moves incrementally, but nonetheless argue for comprehensive change. They believe that by arguing for comprehensive change they pose countervailing power to those who want to preserve the status quo. They believe that incrementalism is possible only as the result of compromise between those who resist any change and those (like they) who argue for total change.

The issue of comprehensive versus incremental change is one of strategy, but also one of tactics. It requires an assessment not only of what might be desirable, but of what is possible at this time and in the foreseeable future, not in some never-never land, but here in the United States.

The second issue that requires debate involves the appropriate role for employers. As already noted, most private health insurance is linked to employment. Medicare and Medicaid are public programs that have broken that link. Nevertheless, for the last forty years, major federal legislative and executive branch proposals to cover all Americans have relied on an expansion of insurance through employment rather than an expansion of Medicare's social insurance approach. The most comprehensive approach to universal coverage would sever the relationship between employment and health insurance.[14] Removing health insurance from the fringe benefit agenda would enhance price competition between employers since they would no longer face health insurance premium payments that depend on the age of their employees, the proportion of early retirees who remain on the firm's health insurance rolls, and the relative costs of medical care in the particular community.

Conversely, there are those who suggest that removing the employer from the picture and substituting government as the "insurer" would require a massive redirecting of dollars now flowing through the system and substantial increases in taxes (albeit offset by declines in private payment). This argument states that the mandating approach was not chosen as the preferred method for trivial or accidental reasons, but in recognition of the complexity involved in changing the flow of funds, the fractious impact on labor negotiations even if only in the short run, as employers and employees tried to "capture" the dollars that had been spent on health insurance, and the deeply held views, shared by many Americans, about the avoidance of additional taxes.

A third issue involves the role of private insurance companies. Since any universal insurance system would involve administrative tasks (for example, those related to payment of providers), some analysts would argue that a "war" against private insurers is a war that need not be fought. They would argue that it is vital to reduce private insurance political opposition to the program and that it therefore is politically useful to have private insurers participate in administering the universal program rather than having it handled entirely by a government agency. In their view, while this might increase program costs, that would be a price worth paying. They might even be willing to permit commercial insurers to retain the underwriting function if we had proper risk adjustment and could adjust premiums so that insurers would not gain by selecting lower-risk subscribers.

Such analysts would suggest that, even if risk adjustment or effective open enrollment were not possible, many insurers might be pleased to retain the opportunity to perform administrative tasks while disengaging from the underwriting and risk-bearing aspects of insurance. It is clear that preserving a role for insurers would displease many who would prefer to rely exclusively on government. It is also clear that having a program akin to Medicare, a program in which reimbursements and payments are administered by organizations and firms in the private sector, but in which government assumes the underwriting role (by enrolling virtually everyone) would be a significant advance over the present situation and more efficient. The appropriate role for private insurers is no trivial decision. It requires evaluation of the political and economic benefits and costs of the various alternatives and extensive debate.

A fourth issue involves the role of for-profit entities in the delivery of medical care. We have indicated that we believe that the expansion of the for-profit sector in health care delivery, the values it has introduced and represents, has been detrimental to those who seek care, to those who deliver it, and to their mutual relationship. Yet the new ethos exists, as do the new attitudes that have come into play. In important ways they reflect our culture at the beginning of the twenty-first century and are not merely dependent on the legal status of a few institutions and facilities. It is difficult to imagine that at this time one could recapture the values of an earlier period and do more than contain the expansion of the for-profit sector, and so we expect that, both in the short and intermediate run, for-profits are here to stay.

Furthermore, it seems clear that at the present time the not-for-profit and/or the public sector do not have the resources for a "buyout" that would compensate private sector stockholder owners of for-profits. Perhaps, in due course, a number of for-profits will leave the field of health care delivery, preferring to devote their energies and resources to other arenas in which they will find a higher rate of return on investment dollars. Perhaps some for-profit entities would find reason to sell one or more of their facilities and identify not-for-profit buyers willing and able to buy. If the federal deficit is cut substantially and the opportunity to have a phased buyout of (parts of) the for-profit sector arises, it will be useful to consider the benefits and costs of for-profit to not-for-profit conversions. In the interim it would be more than helpful to recognize that one cannot simply turn back the clock. One's energies would be usefully spent developing mechanisms that contain further for-profit expansion, that hold for-profits accountable, that induce behaviors that are consonant with social needs, and that generate sufficient resources to achieve those ends.

As the debate over the characteristics of a universal health insurance program is joined, attention should and will be directed to the question of "choice." Some hold that just as competition is a plus, and even more competition is better, so it is with choice. One cannot deny that choice is a valuable thing and that persons want to have choice where choice is relevant. Nevertheless, there is growing evidence that "too many options can result in paralysis, not liberation."[15] This is not meant to suggest that a system without any choice would be desirable. It does suggest, however, that a menu of unconstrained choices may be dysfunctional and reduce rather than increase satisfaction. The appropriate kinds and number of insurance and provider choices that are offered need to be seriously considered. This is especially the case because choices that are offered in a governmentally sponsored or financed program carry an implicit seal of approval in regard to quality, if not value per dollar. If government offers a plan that provides for a particular insurance option or a particular HMO and group of physicians, it must devote the resources necessary to ascertain and monitor the quality of performance. Choice without requisite information to inform decisions is a sham, if not a fraud.

Structuring Universal Health Insurance: A Single Payer Approach

We believe that the most effective, efficient, and equitable health care insurance system would be what has come to be termed (quite inexactly, to be sure) "single payer."[16] It is also sometimes described as "Canadian-like," or traditional "Medicare for all," and we shall use these three terms interchangeably in the ensuing discussion.[17] Such a program would embody a social insurance approach; its financing would rely on (general or earmarked) tax revenues. Its appeal lies in its enrollment simplicity and financing efficiency: as in Medicare, everyone is enrolled and the program is funded through taxation. Recognizing, however, that in the past such a plan has faced political difficulties, we also present an alternative that is more complex because it relies on multiple ways to enroll the covered population, but that nonetheless over time would enable us to attain the goal of universal coverage and preserve the main elements of social cohesion and progressivity that would be obtained in a social insurance program.

The advantage of a single payer system is that it would make insurance truly universal and not dependent on age, employment, residence, income, or other demographic or socioeconomic variables. Only with true universality and the assurance of continued universal coverage can we achieve administrative simplicity, provide insurance to those who today are not covered or are inadequately covered, and remove the fear that now grips many Americans who do have insurance, but who are concerned that they might lose it. While it is true that one can conceive of a scheme in which insurance would be provided to all through a varied menu of programs tailored to individual groups within the larger society, that approach is complicated and inefficient and inevitably threatens the continuity of insurance and of care.

We must ask what the "error rate" would be in a system that would require sorting individuals and families into the particular mechanisms through which they would be enrolled. How many individuals would be confused and would never enroll, how many individuals would enroll in the "incorrect" program and receive fewer benefits than they are entitled to, how many persons would enroll and find that they had to reenroll when they moved, altered marital status, left the household, or changed employers or economic status? Put simply, how many individuals would be "lost"? We believe that traditional values of equity lead to a goal of universal enrollment and, for reasons of efficiency and comprehensiveness, to a single mechanism for enrollment. In turn, that requires a system that is administered and financed by government (or by an institution set up by government and operating in a quasi-governmental manner).

This, we suggest, is more than a matter of redistribution. Redistribution can be achieved in many different ways and does not require a single payer approach. Rather, a "Medicare for all" program is justified by the need for efficiency in enrollment and the criterion of universality. Such a program would not be targeted solely to those most in need and therefore would enroll more individuals than if it were concerned with a low-income subset of the total population. That, however, does not mean that the program would necessarily require a larger or more costly administrative capacity. Indeed, a universal program would demand much less administrative capacity, and, as a corollary, lower administrative expenditures, than a program that, like Medicaid, would involve an ever-changing population and repeated reenrollment.[18]

A universal program that covered everyone who interacted with the health care system could emphasize regionalization and rationalization of health care delivery as well as reduction of administrative and advertising expenditures and waste, thus helping to reduce the long-term rate of increase in expenditures. That explains why estimates of the costs of such universal programs have generally projected a modest rise in health delivery expenditures in the first few years and an early "crossover point" where expenditures under the universal plan would first equal and then be less than projected expenditures under a "status quo" arrangement (with millions of uninsured).

We believe the arguments in favor of a universal social insurance program are powerful. Nevertheless, the history of efforts to achieve universality forces us to recognize that no approach such as the one described here has been advocated (or seriously considered) by the leadership in either of the two major parties since the early 1970s. Furthermore, many of those who led the fight for a tax-based social insurance approach to universal coverage have modified their views. They may still believe that a single payer model is "best," but they do not believe that it is realistic to assume that such a proposal could gain the support of a President, 51 members of the Senate (or more if there were a filibuster), and 218 members of the House. While we respect those who continue to argue for a "Medicare for all" answer and do not negate the contribution they make to the articulation of important values, we feel that political reality compels us to ask whether there are not other ways, even if more complex and more costly, of reaching the goal of health care coverage for all Americans. We believe the answer to that question is yes.

Moreover, the argument against a single payer system does not rest entirely on the absence of the necessary political support. Political support is not something gained and lost through a process akin to winning or losing a lottery. We must ask what lies behind its absence. Why did President Clinton refer to the efficiency of and savings under a Canadian-like system, and then opt for a different approach? What is it that has caused so many to state that "a Medicare-like approach would be preferable, *but . . .* ?" Why do they feel that they would not be able to mount a successful political campaign that would convince the skeptics?

The answer lies in part in the lack of involvement by the kind of citizen groups that pressed for Medicare over a sustained period of time. Over the last four decades there have been a number of proposals for national health insurance, yet after the defeat (or neglect) each suffered, it disappeared from the national agenda and was no longer the subject of debate. Who of us can describe the proposals by President Carter or by Senator Kennedy in the late 1970s or of President Clinton only a little over a decade ago? Why has the necessary infrastructure for sustained efforts at education, political involvement, and legislation about universal insurance not been present?

It is of course true that the political potency of insurance companies and of for-profits in the health arena has grown over the years. This and the campaign contributions provided by individuals, institutions, organizations, firms, and trade associations with a stake in the status quo have proven exceedingly influential and important. Nevertheless, we believe that other factors are also at play. The failure to mobilize resources around national health insurance (and especially around the single payer approach) can be explained somewhat by the fact that legislators shy away from measures that require the imposition of new taxes. Analysts may conclude that national health insurance would not appreciably increase health care expenditures (and that the relatively small increase that would occur would be a short-term phenomenon). Nevertheless, many (perhaps most) people do not believe that and/or fear the distributional impact of the new taxation. The debate about Medicare and its tax implications came at a different time in our economic and political history. In more recent years the litany about government ineptitude and waste, and the accompanying antitax rhetoric, has affected the nature of the debates about health insurance (and other social programs).

Furthermore, the implementation of Medicare did not reorganize the nature of the insurance held by (and thus represent a threat to) the vast majority of Americans. The organized constituency for Medicare was aided by the financial and political resources of a strong labor movement. In contrast, a single payer program, while of great assistance to millions without insurance (and to others), would change the nature of insurance even for that part of the more affluent population that already has, what they believe to be, adequate financial protection.[19] Not certain that they would be better off under the new program, they do not represent an obvious constituency that could be organized and supported without far more effort and resources than could be made available by a now much-weakened labor movement.

In addition to these obstacles legislators are wary of a program that would require a massive shift in the flow of funds that at present move from employers and employees to insurers, and that would have to be redirected into government tax coffers. This redirection would necessarily have a very substantial immediate impact on labor negotiations and collective bargaining, wages, and levels of compensation. Major parts of the organized labor movement have developed comprehensive health benefit packages for their members and have a vested interest in health care as part of collective bargaining (and, in some cases, in operating the health and welfare funds that are part of the collective bargaining agreement).[20] They may not be willing to jeopardize what they already have. Since enactment of a single payer program would have significant distributional impacts, labor leaders would expect assurance that their members would not be harmed by the change.

Beyond all these concerns is the awareness by all involved in legislative efforts that, once passed, the act of legislation is likely to differ markedly from the bill that was initially proposed. That is the nature of our system. The fear is real that early support for a "sensible" program will prove itself an error because the favored program will be changed beyond recognition as it makes its way through committees, debates in both the House and Senate, amendments, and reconciliation between the two chambers. The complications and frustrations of the legislative process serve as yet another obstacle to the enactment of a single payer, tax-based (or, for that matter, any comprehensive) approach.[21]

The recognition of these various impediments has forced us to examine whether a "Medicare for all" approach must be considered as an "all or nothing" proposition with inviolate characteristics, whether something less than a total single payer package can be effective and beneficial. We conclude that one can develop a construct that, though less efficient than a single payer program, could cover all Americans. Furthermore, we are aware that whatever is enacted will inevitably change and evolve over time, and thus, if well designed initially, may develop in ways that bring it closer to a single tax-based social insurance program.

Structuring Universal Insurance: An Incremental Approach

Many "compromises" can be made in designing a program. Given the number of specific issues that need to be addressed in a universal health insurance program, a large number of permutations and combinations are possible.[22] We will not undertake a full examination of the various possibilities, but will offer a road map that we believe could prove useful. It addresses the issue of comprehensiveness versus incrementalism, the role of the federal government versus other avenues for public accountability, mechanisms for funding coverage, and the role of insurance companies.

PHASING

The first compromise that is likely to prove necessary is the phasing in of the program over a period of time. We recognize that possibility even in spite of our belief that the fiscal impact of a universal program would not be unduly large. Nevertheless, given the state of the American economy, the size of the current and prospective deficit, and other social needs, we anticipate that it would be difficult (politically, if not economically) to move to universal coverage in a single step. A program that would cover all those without insurance and, furthermore, provide comprehensive benefits for all whose coverage is inadequate may be too much for the body politic. Moreover, though the national fiscal impact of such a program may be "reasonable," the distributive aspects (by region, industry, and firm) might be considerable.

At the same time it should be clear that it would be most unfortunate to postpone action that would provide insurance to some who today are uninsured and wait for the optimum moment when we are able to cover the entire population all at once. Medicare did not initially cover all the aged population nor did it add the disabled until the 1973 amendments; similarly, Medicaid did not cover all the poor, and the State Children's Health Insurance Program (SCHIP) did not provide insurance to every child without it. But the fact that we should have done better does not invalidate the contribution that these programs have made. Millions of individuals are better off because of them and the companion state programs than they would be without them. Indeed, we would argue that all of us (whether or not we are enrolled in any of these programs) are better off as a result.

We believe that a phased approach that could be considered as a logical step from which other steps would follow (not something that would be "temporary," that is, repealed and replaced at some later date) is a responsible course of action. While it is true that a phased approach would mean that some Americans would not enter the program till a second or third or even later phase became effective, our judgment is that the various phases, including the final one, would result in the attainment of universal coverage earlier than would be the case if supporters of universal coverage insisted that everything be done in one step and continued to wait for that step to be taken.

The traditional argument against phasing has been that it would require revisiting and debating the extension of insurance coverage every time a new stage is proposed. As a consequence the political process would be forced to reinitiate and renew the insurance debate again, and again, and again. However, the phasing process can be designed another way: it can instead entail a set of stages, spelled out in advance and embodied in the legislation. These stages could have trigger mechanisms that would delay or advance implementation, but whatever happens would happen automatically. This is not a concept that is unknown to the body politic. While it is true that a future Congress could change the legislation and the timetable, it would require congressional action as well as a Presidential signature to do so. That is very different than a phasing approach that requires that every future

Congress again enter into debate before any action be taken. To enact a program that becomes fully effective over a period of time is very different from enacting one step, then, with no date certain, leaving it to the future to discuss, debate, and enact the next one. We believe that to insist on nothing less than "everything" is to carry rigidity to an extreme.

There are only a limited number of ways that enrollment in a program can be phased in. One can do so, for example, by income, by state, by age, and by uninsured/insured status. We do not believe that using income as an enrollment determinant (in a sense, a better version of Medicaid) moves us toward universality. Generally the argument in favor of a phasing method focused on those with lowest income is that assistance would be targeted to those who are most needy. The argument against it is also clear: it maintains a "welfare" approach, does not build a strong constituency for the next step, sets no real precedent for action toward universality, and does not create a program that can evolve, or be seen as evolving, into something more comprehensive and more efficient.

Furthermore, using income as a criterion would perpetuate one of the more problematic characteristics of the existing Medicaid program: the need to check income and to disenroll and reenroll individuals as their incomes change, inevitably adding to administrative complexity and costs. Would an expansion of funds that would enable Medicaid to extend its eligibility be useful? Of course it would, and especially so since the budget crises in the various states in the last few years have led to significant cutbacks in that program. Such an expansion, however, would do little to move us any closer to the goal of universal coverage. "Expanding Medicaid" is not synonymous with "the first step toward universal insurance."

A phasing method that involves putting a program in place a few states at a time—for example, five states a year over a period of ten years, or ten a year for a period of five years—adds complexity to a health care system that needs rationalization and simplicity. Given the number of national firms or firms that operate in more than one state, a staggered approach would create administrative difficulties for businesses that provide insurance to their employees. Furthermore, the mobility of the American population would create additional complexity since individuals who have insurance at a particular time might lose their coverage if they relocated to a state that had not yet been phased into the program. The changing residence characteristics of individuals as they moved from eligibility to ineligibility, and perhaps back again, produce a variant of the income problem already noted, without the redeeming virtue of providing aid to the neediest among us.

In contrast with income or residence as enrollment criteria, phasing by age, we believe, does show considerable merit. Many proponents who view Medicare's age standard as a building block toward universality have considered additional blocks that would fill in the ages up to sixty-five. This could be accomplished either by lowering the age eligibility (for Medicare or its equivalent) in successive steps or by enrolling children and raising the coverage age till it reached sixty-five. An approach that uses age to phase in the program is "logical" and makes clear that the goal is universality. It has the additional virtue (as with Medicare for those sixty-five and over) that an age determinant for eligibility is easily administered—eligibility does not require continuous reexamination and recertification. Furthermore, this phasing method easily meets the requirement that the program expand "automatically" and not be dependent on the enactment of additional legislation at each stage.

Historically, any expansion of Medicare that begins with children has garnered more support than one whose approach is to start by reducing the eligibility age below sixty-five. Indeed, there have been numerous proposals for creating the equivalent of Medicare for children ("Kiddycare" was one suggested name). Because children generally have a low rate of hospitalization, per capita expenditures on behalf of children's health are not very high. In the year 2000, for example, per person health spending in the age group 0–5 was $1,525 (and about the same in the age groups 5–14 and 15–24). As one would expect, spending increases with age, and is over $9,000 per person in the age group 65–74.[23] Thus many more children can be enrolled for the same number of dollars as would be true for persons in older age groups. The consequent added visibility of the program could prove politically beneficial.

In addition, given the sums already available through SCHIP (as well as through employer/employee health insurance coverage), many children could be covered with only a modest increase in national health expenditures. If one begins with children and selects appropriate phasing sequences and time intervals, no child covered in one time period would lose coverage as he or she aged. Additionally, the age in the initial phase and in subsequent phases could be selected in a manner that (by selecting unequal age intervals) distributes the fiscal impact in fairly equal increments year by year as the program moves forward. Thus, for example, one might cover all children up to age 18 in year one, add twelve years extending the program to those age 30 and below in year two, to 40 in year three, to 48 in year four, 55 in year five, 61 in year six, and 65 in the seventh year. It is clear that there are a very large number of possible combinations that would begin with children, increase eligibility age so that the child would not lose coverage as he or she aged, and include the entire population within a limited period of time. Indeed, one can combine a children's program with a reduction of the Medicare age of sixty-five, thus covering the extremely vulnerable group of early voluntary and involuntary retirees.

Yet one more phasing approach would initiate the program by enrolling the uninsured. We do not discuss that proposal here; instead, the problem of the uninsured will be addressed within our comments on the structural aspects of the universal program—how persons are enrolled, what they are enrolled in, how the program is funded. These issues need to be faced whatever phasing approach is selected, and are the subjects to which we now turn.

ENROLLMENT AND FINANCING

Having stated that phasing can begin by covering a particular demographic group (such as children), we must address the question of how they would be covered, that is, through what mechanism and by what organized entity. As our model we look to the medical insurance program that already exists for federal employees, retirees, and their dependents, the Federal Employees Health Benefits (FEHB) program, which covers nine million persons. In that program, private fee-for-service insurers and organized delivery systems (such as HMOs) offer their packages at various premiums and (if approved) enroll those federally covered individuals who elect that particular insurer or delivery system. The insurer is required to accept all individuals who apply (the standard "open enrollment" requirement).

Thus private sector organizations compete for enrollees. Government is not the provider of care, but the organizer of the market and convener of participants. It is true that an arrangement that presumes the continued presence of insurers (not merely as bill payers, but as underwriters) is fraught with difficulties: if, as at the present time, there are no risk adjustments, insurers may attempt to "game" the system, that is, enroll the healthiest individuals. Because of wider differences in health status, this is likely to be a more severe problem for the unemployed (and others) than is the case in the FEHB program, which covers federal employees, a diverse and, yet, more homogeneous group. This fundamental problem is avoided when, as in Medicare, there is only one insurer, and everyone, by definition, is in the same group. In a new FEHB-like program the real question is whether "correct" risk adjustment is possible and whether one can rely on strong federal oversight. Since we feel that it would be difficult to exclude the private insurance sector without providing the opportunity for participation, we would rely on such risk adjustment as is possible and on strong monitoring of open enrollment and accountability.[24] We are convinced that it would be politically much easier to alter program characteristics if insurers do not perform as they should, than to exclude them entirely from the program without recourse to experience and evidence about their behavior.

Over the long run we believe it would be useful to encourage an arm's-length relationship between insurance companies and HMO and other managed care deliverers. We would recommend that the program include provisions (and funding) that over time would enable not-for-profit groups (including care providers) to take over (on a voluntary basis and with appropriate compensation) delivery organizations now controlled by for-profit insurers, and would urge that these not-for-profit entities expand the degree of consumer representation and authority on boards. While consumer representation and not-for-profit status do not guarantee appropriate behavior (and especially so in a competitive market), we believe they do increase its probability.

The approach outlined, using the federal employees' program as a model, can easily be adapted to yet one other alternative phasing approach. Thus, for example, rather than beginning with children,[25] one could start by enrolling the 45 million Americans who are uninsured, with government paying all or part of the premium, depending on individual or family income.[26] Indeed, the program could have a very substantial impact if it began by enrolling the uninsured, Medicaid recipients, Medicare beneficiaries, and other individuals with federally financed coverage into a single FEHB program.[27] Such an approach would aid tens of millions of individuals (in itself a worthwhile goal) and would do so in a manner that would create a program strong enough to set standards, monitor quality, and address health care delivery issues that extend beyond the financial aspects of insurance costs and program benefits. This would have a very substantial impact on the creation of performance guidelines and administrative procedures for the entire health care system. The potential enrollment could include 45 million uninsured (and many more if those who are uninsured for brief periods of time are included), perhaps an equal number of the inadequately insured, some 45 million Medicaid recipients, over 40 million Medicare beneficiaries, and about 9 million federal employees, a potential total of over 175 million subscribers (which is roughly equal to the 175 million individuals—including many inadequately insured—who have employer-assisted health insurance). Though not universal, such a program would be large and strong enough (especially if it included members of Congress and federal employees) to assure that it would not be weakened over time.

It would also be appropriate to permit individuals (including those with employer-provided health insurance coverage) to enroll in the new program—with appropriate individual and/or employer contributions—if they preferred to receive care from an organization within that entity.[28] Such a provision would enable individuals who had been enrolled in the federal program to maintain continuity with their former medical provider if their employment status changed and their new employer's health insurance package did not include enrollment in the managed care organization to which the individual belonged while in the FEHB program. Similarly, the opportunity to stay with or join FEHB would enable provider continuity for individuals who change employers or who move in and out of employment. Importantly, the competition between the federal enrollment program and other ways of entering the insurance market would provide real-time information on the strengths and weaknesses in the various insurance plans. Building on competition, such an approach would enable the FEHB program (or its equivalent) to become a virtual single payer mechanism if, over time, enough subscribers chose it. It would become the single payer of claims even for individuals enrolled through different employers and with payments flowing in from different sources.

The creation of a new federally funded program that would exist in the presence of privately funded employer programs would necessarily raise difficult issues, all of them requiring some kind of resolution. What of those employees whose employer-provided health insurance benefits are not as comprehensive as those provided under the new federal program—would there be an incentive for employers to drop coverage for their employees who might then become eligible for federal coverage, and what should be done about such matters? Would early retirees be enrolled in the new program, or should the age for Medicare enrollment be lowered to accommodate such individuals? We mention these issues (the list of possibilities that such a program would raise and that would require ex-ante resolution is, of course, much longer) in order to illustrate the fact that any program that is less than fully comprehensive and less than fully universal and that relies upon a phasing approach inevitably involves complex interrelationships with already existing insurance mechanisms.

Rejection of the single payer initiative—under which these questions would not arise—means that one must face the kinds of issues we have just outlined. Nevertheless, many of those challenges are of a temporary nature, and all of them can be solved. They need to be viewed as problems to be addressed rather than, as so often has been the case in past debates about extending health insurance, as obstacles that are insurmountable and that provide an excuse for not taking action. Complexities are and always will be present: the health sector is almost 15 percent of the American economy, and restructuring it, even with a universal and comprehensive social insurance program, must involve complicated (but fixable) transition issues. Nevertheless, the various issues can be anticipated, solutions can be developed, and the concerns can be resolved. Indeed, we can guarantee that in a world of scientific discoveries and medical innovations, and, moreover, in one of changing economic relationships and demographic patterns—in other words, in the real and ever-changing world we live in—new issues will emerge, new problems will occur, and yesterday's approaches will need to be adapted. One is fundamentally in error if one imagines that there is a universal health insurance "solution" that can be set in place without expectation of further adjustment.

The expansion of existing programs to cover a cohort of children (or the uninsured) would require new federal expenditures. That, of course, has also been the case for any of the various health insurance programs that have been proposed over the last thirty years, including those that mandated coverage by employers but had to subsidize employers and employees whose profits and wages were too low to absorb the new mandated costs. All programs that would expand coverage need to be financed and, depending on the structure of the program, some or all of that financing must come from government. If the program is to be budget-neutral, expenditures in other areas (many of high priority) must be reduced, or the necessary funds must be raised through general or earmarked taxes. Raising new government dollars needs to be done in a progressive fashion (that is, with the amount of assistance toward the purchase of health insurance or toward enrollment in a health plan inversely related to income). It is clear that the new funds cannot be obtained solely from those newly covered since, in general, those individuals and families have below-average incomes.

Health care (like education) for all necessarily calls for redistribution. Those who oppose additional redistribution of the tax burden are implicitly opposed to providing health insurance (or, indeed, sufficient health care) to the uninsured, most of whom are low-income individuals. However, the nature of the appropriate tax mechanism and of its level does not lie at the heart of the proposal we offer. Those are issues that would have to be resolved, but belong in another venue, one that is in command of the most recent Department of the Treasury and Census Bureau data, that can subject those data to rigorous analysis, and that can consider the health insurance tax burden in relation to other taxes that are levied by local, state, and federal government. That is not the task before us. There also would need to be a redistribution of real resources (additional personnel and facilities) in areas that are underserved. As we have pointed out, this will require a planning policy and support for interventions such as community health centers (and satellite hospitals in a regional plan).[29]

PROGRAM ADMINISTRATION AND COST CONTAINMENT

Finally, we turn to a description of the structure for administration of the insurance program and of the various health care delivery system issues, such as educational assistance, planning, and capital expansion, that were discussed earlier. In doing so, we recognize that the terms "single payer," "Medicare for all," and even "Canadian-like" all conjure up an image of federal government administration.[30] There is little question that many Americans are fearful that the kind of program described here would put very substantial powers in the hands of "Washington." Even with the best of motivations, such power can be abused, and history suggests that we cannot always rely on the best of motivations.

Given these attitudes toward Washington, the efforts within a few states to move toward universal coverage may pose a promising alternative. One might be tempted to assign the responsibility for health insurance reform to the individual states while providing "carrots" and "sticks" (rewards and penalties) to encourage each state to design, implement, and administer its own program and mechanism designed to attain such coverage. Indeed, Dr. Fein first made just such a proposal almost two decades ago.[31] A "federalist" approach that views the states as "laboratories," however, cannot negate the important regulatory and fiscal role that must be played by the federal government. Federal regulators would have to make certain that each state achieved universal coverage and such other conditions as the enabling legislation required. Furthermore, given the wide economic disparities among the states, significant funding responsibility would necessarily rest with the federal government. We need Washington.

We also need the other levels of government. As noted, the health care delivery system (not only the health care financing system) must change, and that change will encompass greater planning, regionalization, and rationalization. Given the size and diversity of the United States, such efforts cannot be effectively conducted only in, or emanate only from, Washington. We need levels of administration below Washington, and envision a network both of national and regional boards. We believe that a national quasi-governmental nonpartisan commission (analogous to the Board of Governors of the Federal Reserve System) should be formed with responsibilities to administer the federal health insurance system and to recommend levels of funding and of insurance benefits to Congress.[32] It would receive the private and public funds for coverage for those who would be enrolled in the system that it administers and disburse payments to insurers on behalf of those enrollees. In addition, it would be charged with the responsibility to monitor, evaluate, and take such actions as would be necessary to improve the quality of care. Finally, it would have the responsibility to implement measures to reduce both public and private administrative expenses by developing standard insurance, enrollment, billing, and electronic claims-processing forms.

The major responsibilities for planning health care delivery system changes should be integrated with actions by the regional boards (analogous to the regional Federal Reserve banks) that would be created coterminous with the existing regional structures of the Department of Health and Human Services and of Medicare and Medicaid (through the Centers for Medicare and Medicaid Services), which divide the fifty states into ten regions.[33] Since the United States Public Health Service is organized through the same regions, an insurance and planning system administered with geographically similar regional offices would be able to integrate the responsibilities for medical care and for public health activities.

We are convinced that cost containment requires more than rhetoric and "jaw-boning" and more than the (sometimes heroic) efforts by individual institutions and other participants in the delivery of care. Imperative as planning is, its implementation necessitates budgetary controls. We would require that the regional authorities develop projected or recommended health care operating and capital budgets and that these be transmitted to the central board. In turn, those budgets would provide the basis for the development of a national operating and capital budget (which, subsequently, would be allocated into final regional budgets). This budget should include support that is sufficient to generate and regenerate workforce resources (including support for medical education). The development of budgets would provide opportunity for debate about mechanisms, opportunities, and meaningful trade-offs to restrain medical care inflation and expenditures, and ultimately about appropriate levels of funding.

In arguing that budgetary control is necessary, we emphasize that the purpose of a budget is to raise questions about trade-offs. The United States is a rich country, and the new opportunities in the field of medicine are great. Therefore, it may be that citizens would collectively determine that they desire to spend an increasing proportion of the GDP on national health expenditures (including disease prevention and health promotion as well as acute interventions). It is important that we understand what we are giving up in order to increase (or maintain) health care spending. It is also important that we understand the price we pay for inefficiencies and waste. A budget would necessitate that we focus on those kinds of issues.

We recognize that such debates are not only about what might be considered "technical" matters. Nevertheless, we believe that it would be useful to insulate, insofar as possible, the boards from the heavy dose of partisanship that could jeopardize their activities. To that end we would urge that the terms of office, selection, and approval of board members and regional administrators should follow procedures designed to maximize the nonpartisan character of their various supervisory and policy responsibilities. Furthermore, we believe that there must be significant representation and input from the general public, and therefore recommend that a substantial proportion of central and regional board members be nonprofessionals in the health field, that they be selected as individuals who represent the public, and that mechanisms be developed to facilitate substantial public input.

Although we have indicated that the national board should receive the funds provided on behalf of the individuals covered through the FEHB mechanism, the board need not be expected to set up a mechanism for collecting said sums. Such a mechanism already exists. Efficiency would be enhanced by using the Internal Revenue Service (IRS) as the "collection" agency for premiums. While it is true that the IRS is not generally perceived as a "friendly" agency, it has the competence to perform this function. Furthermore, since it has information on the income of individuals and household units, it is in a position to administer a system that varies the premium in relation to income. It can easily make the system progressive by varying a credit against taxes that is dependent on the health insurance premium and the individual's income, and by providing a payment (the equivalent of a "negative income tax") to those at the lowest income who do not owe taxes (or taxes that are less than the premium credit they are due).[34]

We should also note an important feature of the IRS: one could build on its traditional role of fiscal agent in collecting revenues, including Social Security and Medicare payroll taxes, enabling us to move away from employment-based health insurance. That historical accident has been the source of much mischief. It has made the achievement of universality more rather than less difficult by requiring that mandated plans monitor changes in employment and wages and provide subsidies, exemptions, and special programs for those without employment, and therefore inhibiting true competition around issues of productivity rather than hiring policies. It would not be administratively difficult for the IRS to handle what can be considered a refundable (and progressive) tax credit that would mesh with the newly expanded federal employee insurance program, with private employer insurance, and with individual payment. The degree of assistance for the purchase of insurance would be dependent on income, and the subsidy could range from 100 percent of the cost of insurance at the lowest incomes to zero percent (or some minimal amount) at the highest.[35]

It is important to note that the structure that we describe (the use of the Federal Employees Health Benefits Program) together with the IRS tax mechanism provides an administratively simple way to achieve universality through, for example, a requirement that every individual purchase insurance (with an appropriate subsidy to enable that purchase), thus breaking the link to employment in one step.[36] Alternatively, if necessary, one could adopt a phased approach. One could envision a plan in which children, or the uninsured, Medicaid recipients, or others, entered into the federal program, and all other Americans could similarly choose that option (or any other plan that met federal specifications for the benefits provided). Everyone would be required to purchase insurance, but those who needed assistance to do so would receive it (including, at very low incomes, a refund for the full cost of the insurance).

Such a tax-credit non-employment-based program would replace existing "tax expenditures," the tax benefit provided to those individuals whose employers pay for their health insurance, and who are not required to pay taxes on those premium payments. While many persons would find that the loss of today's benefit would be made up for by the federal IRS refundable tax credit, there would be some higher-income individuals whose tax benefit gains were above average and who would lose more than they otherwise gained. In general, it is clear that the greater the progressivity and redistribution, the greater the losses by persons at the top of the income ladder. Who would win and who would lose, and how much would be won or lost, would depend on the level of assistance the plan provided and the marginal tax bracket that the individual faced.

The course we have outlined builds on familiar arrangements: phasing (by age or by insurance status), creating a federal program that extends the FEHB program already in place, and providing federal financial assistance that would enable individuals to enroll in the new program, thus making it possible for individuals who have no employer or employer-provided insurance to acquire coverage. It would preserve a (limited) role for insurance companies and managed care entities. We do not imply that these various approaches would be acceptable to all parties: some would want to move more rapidly (even if it meant paying more taxes) while others would not want to move at all (preferring no increase in expenditures or taxes); some would not want insurers to play any underwriting or administrative role while others would want them to retain the roles they now play; and some would want to eliminate the employer-linked insurance mechanism while others would object to the creation of a large (though not all-inclusive) tax-based federal program.

As with many of the characteristics of social programs (including universal health insurance), what seems difficult to visualize is often so because, caught up in ideological rhetoric, there is a focus on disagreements rather than on agreements, on why things can't work rather than how to make them work. We do not believe that we can achieve a more equitable health care system without universal coverage. More to the point, we do not believe that the achievement of universal coverage in the United States is a matter of finding solutions to puzzling technical issues. The solutions exist. They have been implemented in other countries (though each country has its own unique plan), and researched, proposed, written about, and debated here. Various proposals may offer a somewhat new wrinkle, a new way to administer the program, a new way to phase it in, and thereby (because of the many variables and possible combinations) create a proposal that appears to be "new."

Nevertheless, the major options and contours are well known: there are only so many ways to expand the insurance pool and enroll newly insured individuals, only so many ways to finance the expansion of services, only so many administrative control possibilities. The problem is not that we have not completed yet another set of studies; the problem is not that we lack knowledge. Rather, solving the problem of universal coverage requires finding a way to reconcile contrasting views about the role of the market and of government, of competition and of planning, of individualism and of community. In our judgment America has the needed research base and social strategy. What remains necessary is to generate the political will to persevere in the quest for a more equitable health care system. A first step toward that end is a renewal of the discussion about the need for a universal program. It is once again time to do so.[37]

The medical agenda of the United States is long, rich, and challenging. As our review of the last century demonstrates, so it has been and, we believe, will continue to be. Over the twentieth century we have witnessed an educational, scientific, consumer, regulatory, and entrepreneurial revolution. We expect that during the twenty-first century medicine's and public health's abilities to treat patients and improve the quality of life, to prevent disease, and to promote health will expand far beyond what we might have imagined only a few years ago. We believe that medicine's scientific advances have to be matched by advances in its organization and financing. We are convinced that if we apply ourselves, we can make significant progress toward that goal early in this century.

We recognize that the health care system is part of society, both reflecting and affecting the society it serves. Thus we cannot expect to achieve universal insurance without a collective decision that our value system calls for equity and that we are prepared to take the necessary redistributive actions to achieve it. As we have indicated, even a limited perspective that focuses solely on health advancement requires examination of (and action in) housing, nutrition, economic status, employment, and the environment, among other areas. Universal health insurance and access and promotion of health, therefore, are more than matters of health policy. In a fundamental sense they are matters of social policy and require a social revolution.

Yet we will find that when that social revolution takes place, we will move on to another set of challenging and pressing issues. This should not surprise us, for as long as a society is changing—and an alive and vibrant society will always be in flux—so, too, will medicine and its socioeconomic arrangements. Our challenge will be to anticipate those changes so that all Americans can share in the benefits of our scientific progress.

Notes

Introduction

1. Both of us have written books that address some of the matters discussed in this volume. See Julius B. Richmond, *Currents in American Medicine: A Developmental View of Medical Care and Education* (Cambridge, Mass.: Harvard University Press, 1969), and Rashi Fein, *Medical Care, Medical Costs: The Search for a Health Insurance Policy* (Cambridge, Mass.: Harvard University Press, 1986, 1989).

1. The Educational and Scientific Revolution

1. For a more detailed description of this period, see Paul Starr, *The Social Transformation of American Medicine* (New York: Basic Books, 1982).

2. Abraham Flexner, *Medical Education in the United States and Canada* (New York: Carnegie Foundation for the Advancement of Teaching, Bulletin No. 4, 1910). See also T. N. Bonner, *Iconoclast: Abraham Flexner and a Life in Learning* (Baltimore: Johns Hopkins University Press, 2002), for a comprehensive treatment of Flexner's many contributions.

3. Rashi Fein, *The Doctor Shortage: An Economic Diagnosis* (Washington: Brookings Institution, 1967), pp. 66–67. It was some eighty years before the ratio reached the 1906 level.

4. See J. G. Freymann, "Leadership in American Medicine: A Matter of Personal Responsibility," *NEJM* 270, No. 710 (1964), and M. Fishbein, *A History of the American Medical Association 1847–1947: With the Biographies of the Presidents of the Association by Walter A. Bierring: And With Histories of the Publications, Councils, Bureaus, and Other Official Bodies* (Philadelphia: Saunders, 1947).

5. *Medical Care for the American People: The Final Report of the Committee on the Costs of Medical Care,* adopted Oct. 31, 1932 (Chicago: University of Chicago Press, 1932).

6. Committee on the Costs of Medical Care, *Medical Care for the American People* (Chicago: University of Chicago Press, 1932; reprint, U.S. Department of Health, Education, and Welfare, 1970), p. iii.

7. Editorial, *JAMA* 99 (Dec. 3, 1932), p. 1952, as cited in Odin W. Anderson, "Compulsory Medical Care Insurance, 1910–1950," *Medical Care for Americans: Annals of the American Academy of Political and Social Sciences* (January 1951), pp. 106–113.

8. *American Medicine: Expert Testimony out of Court* (New York: The American Foundation, 1937), 2 vols.

9. "The Committee for the Presentation of Certain Principles and Proposals in the Provision of Medical Care," *NEJM* 217, No. 798 (1937).

10. "Editorial: The American Foundation Proposals for Medical Care," *JAMA* 109, No. 1281 (1937).

11. In 1962 the NIH established Institutes concerned with processes rather than organs or diseases (for example, the National Institute of Child Health and Human Development and the National Institute on the General Medical Sciences). Today the NIH has twenty Institutes (including the National Library of Medicine) and seven Centers.

12. Ruth Hanft, "National Health Expenditures, 1950–65," *Social Security Bulletin* 30, No. 3 (February 1967), as cited in Julius B. Richmond, *Currents in American Medicine: A Developmental View of Medical Care and Medical Education* (Cambridge, Mass.: Harvard University Press, 1969), pp. 30, 31.

13. Quoted in *Journal of Medical Education* 42, No. 7 (part 2) (July 1967), pp. 73–74.

14. Quoted in "Biomedical Policy: LBJ's Query Leads to an Illuminating Conference," *Science* 154, No. 619 (Nov. 4, 1966), as cited in Richmond, *Currents in American Medicine*, p. 35.

15. George Packer Berry, dean of Harvard Medical School, was a leader in this effort. See Julius B. Richmond, "Pathsetter in National Pedagogy," *Harvard Medical School Alumni Bulletin* (Spring 1987), p. 35.

16. See Richard Harris, *A Sacred Trust* (New York: New American Library, 1966).

2. The Consumer Revolution

1. Justin F. Kimball, "Prepayment Plan of Hospital Care," *Bulletin of the American Hospital Association* (July 1934), pp. 42–47.

2. Selwyn D. Colins and Clark Tibbets, *Research Memorandum on Social Aspects of Health in the Depression* (New York: Social Science Research Council; reprint, Arno Press, 1972), pp. 146–149.

3. American Medical Association v. United States, and Medical Society of the District of Columbia v. United States, 317 U.S. 519 (1943).

4. American Medical Association v. United States, and Medical Society of the District of Columbia v. United States, 130 F.2d 233, 246 (D.C. Cir. 1942) (notes omitted).

5. See *http://www.greenislandgraphics.com/kp_fujitsu/learn/kphist.html.*

6. RBC Financial Group, "The Insurance Principle and What Insurance Does," *Royal Bank Letter* (April 1972), 53, No. 4, at *http://www.rbc.com/community/letter/april1972.html.*

7. Harry Becker, ed., *Prepayment and the Community,* Report of the Commission on Financing Hospital Care, vol. 2 (New York: McGraw-Hill, 1955), pp. 6, 11.

8. Richard H. Shryock, *The Development of Modern Medicine: An Interpretation of the Social and Scientific Factors Involved* (New York: Alfred A. Knopf, 1936, 1947), p. 384.

9. Ellen Meara, Chapin White, and David M. Cutler, "Trends in Medical Spending, by Age 1963–2000," *Health Affairs* 23, No. 4 (July–August 2004).

10. L. W. Mayo, *A Report of the President's Panel on a Proposed Program for National Action to Combat Mental Retardation* (Washington: U.S. Government Printing Office, 1963).

11. Joint Commission on Mental Illness and Health, *Action for Mental Health: Final Report of the Joint Commission* (New York: Basic Books, 1961).

12. Julius B. Richmond, *Currents in American Medicine: A Developmental View of Medical Care and Medical Education* (Cambridge, Mass.: Harvard University Press, 1969), pp. 70–74.

13. *Comprehensive Neighborhood Health Services Programs* (Washington: Office of Economic Opportunity, 1967).

14. For a rich legislative history of the enactment of Medicare, see such sources as Richard Harris, *A Sacred Trust* (New York: New American Library, 1966); Eugene Feingold, *Medicare: Policy and Politics* (San Francisco: Chandler, 1966); Theodore R. Marmor, *The Politics of Medicare,* 2d ed. (New York: Aldine de Gruyter, 2000); Peter A. Corning, *The Evolution of Medicare: From Idea to Law,* Social Security Administration Research Report No. 29 (Washington: U.S. Government Printing Office, 1969).

15. If the physician charges more than the Medicare-approved fee and does not "take assignment" and receive reimbursement from the Medicare system, the patient would pay the full fee and be reimbursed by Medicare for 80 percent of the approved part.

16. As cited in Irwin Wolkstein, "Medicare 1971: Changing Attitudes and Changing Legislation," *Law and Contemporary Problems* (Autumn 1970), part 2, pp. 697–715.

3. Emerging Tensions between Regulation and Market Forces

1. See Julius B. Richmond, *Currents in American Medicine: A Developmental View of Medical Care and Education* (Cambridge, Mass.: Harvard University Press, 1969), p. 76.

2. See Richard A. Knox, "Doctors Voice Concern over Morality of War," *Boston Globe* (Oct. 14, 1969), as well as a large number of articles published the day after the moratorium, *Boston Globe* (Oct. 16, 1969).

3. Kim Parker, "Dress Code for Medical Students," *NEJM* 293, No. 16 (1975), p. 833; Fitzhugh Mullan, *White Coat, Clenched Fist: The Political Education of an American Physician* (New York: MacMillan, 1976), pp. 20–22.

4. Mullan, *White Coat*, p. 66.

5. As the first director of the national community health centers program during the War on Poverty, Julius Richmond was hardly suspect on the need to expand services to the poor and did not believe in putting aside today's concerns simply in order to create more knowledge or even to create a better world at some point in the distant future. Neither, however, did he feel it was appropriate to ignore the possibility that today's research (even research that seemed "esoteric") might have great favorable implications for those who were in need of help.

6. The Consumer Price Index for all items rose from a base of 100 in 1967 to 170.5 in 1976. Medical care services rose from a base of 100 in 1967 to 197.1 in 1976. *The Annual Report of the Council of Economic Advisers, 1978* (Washington: U.S. Government Printing Office, 1978), pp. 314–315.

7. Calculated from *The Annual Report of the Council of Economic Advisers, 1975* (Washington: U.S. Government Printing Office, 1975), p. 302.

8. See Figure 3 in Chapter 4 for an example of the lack of relationship between health expenditures and health performance in the United States.

9. Conference Report, "Competition in the Health Sector: Past, Present, and Future," Federal Trade Commission (March 1978).

10. The independent practice association (IPA) also defined a set of economic relationships that put the providers of care at financial risk. In an IPA a group of independent physicians continue to practice under fee-for-service arrangements but guarantee to provide medical care to subscribers even if premium revenues prove insufficient to reimburse providers at predetermined fees-for-services. Since physicians continue to practice in their existing locations, IPAs offer familiar arrangements both to physicians and to those individuals whose personal physicians join the IPA panel.

11. A comprehensive review of HMO performance is found in Harold Luft,

Health Maintenance Organizations: Dimensions of Performance (New York: John Wiley & Sons, 1981).

12. The administration did not adopt the consumer control characteristic that Kennedy and others favored.

13. See *http://www.greenislandgraphics.com/kp_fujitsu/learn/kphist.html.*

14. The development of for-profit HMOs and their impact are explored more fully in the next chapter.

15. This became most evident a decade later when, during the debate over the Clinton program, one of the issues that opponents exploited successfully was the constraint on free choice.

16. One of the criticisms sometimes heard about the organization of British hospital care was that one's general physician did not follow the patient into the hospital, leading to a break in continuity of care both when the patient entered and when he or she left the hospital. American continuity of care was a source of pride and considered exceedingly important—till it became less robust.

17. For a rich discussion of HMO performance after 1980, see Robert Miller and Harold Luft, "Managed Care Plan Performance since 1980," *JAMA* 27, No. 19 (1994), pp. 1512–1519, and Robert Miller and Harold Luft, "Does Managed Care Lead to Better or Worse Quality of Care?" *Health Affairs* 16, No. 5 (September–October 1997), pp. 7–25.

18. The House Ways and Means Committee was especially important because tax legislation had to originate in the House. As chairman, Mills was especially powerful because the Committee, most often in the person of Mills, made all the assignments of new members to other committees. Defying the chairman was not encouraged.

19. One article—"110 Handpicked Medical Thinkers Tell You What Will Happen over the Next Five Years," *Medical Economics* (Oct. 29, 1973)—reported that over half of the "experts" consulted believed that the nation would have national health insurance before 1978. An additional 18 percent thought it would happen in 1978.

20. See "National Health Insurance Proposals: Provisions of Bills Introduced in the 93rd Congress as of July 1974," HEW Publication No. (SSA) 75-11920, which lists some twenty different bills. This Publication updated two earlier compilations. See also "National Health Insurance Resource Book," prepared by the staff of the Committee on Ways and Means (Washington: Government Printing Office, 1974).

21. Economists have long argued that employees, not employers, bear the costs of health insurance in the form of lower wages. Nevertheless, many em-

ployers believe that they are the party at risk—and the more so if there were a new financial obligation that could not be financed by an immediate reduction in wages.

22. For a view that the labor movement was less than fully supportive of NHI because it preferred to negotiate benefits on behalf of its members, see Marie Gottschalk, *The Shadow Welfare State: Labor, Business, and the Politics of Health Care in the United States* (Ithaca: Cornell University Press, 2000).

23. This was certainly the case during the Carter presidency. In a 1976 campaign speech at Howard University, candidate Carter advocated national health insurance. By the time he was inaugurated in 1977, the agenda had changed; medical care prices had increased by 10 percent in 1976 and were to increase by an additional 9.9 percent in 1977.

24. It continued to increase and reached 15.5 percent in 2004. See National Center for Health Statistics (NCHS), *Health, United States, 2000, with Adolescent Health Chartbook* (Hyattsville, Md.: NCHS, 2000), Table 115, and Stephen Heffler, "Health Spending Projections through 2013," *Health Affairs*, Web exclusive (Feb. 11, 2004).

25. National Center for Health Statistics, *Health, United States, 1988* (Hyattsville, Md.: NCHS, 1988), Table 115, and *Health, United States, 2003* (Hyattsville, Md.: NCHS, 2003), Table 112.

26. Rashi Fein, *Medical Care, Medical Costs: The Search for a Health Insurance Policy* (Cambridge, Mass.: Harvard University Press, 1986), p. 153.

27. An excellent account exploring these matters during the Roosevelt period can be found in Daniel S. Hirshfield, *The Lost Reform* (Cambridge, Mass.: Harvard University Press, 1970). Similar matters in reference to the battle for Medicare are presented in a gripping fashion in Richard Harris, *A Sacred Trust* (New York: New American Library, 1966).

28. Subcommittee on Health and the Environment of the Committee on Interstate and Foreign Commerce, U.S. House of Representatives, *A Discursive Dictionary of Health Care* (Washington: U.S. Government Printing Office, 1976), p. 106.

29. Statement by Secretary Joseph Califano before the Committee on Finance of the U.S. Senate, March 27, 1979, in *National Health Insurance: Working Papers*, vol. 2 (Washington: U.S. Public Health Service, HEW, n.d.), p. 5.

30. The Committee for National Health Insurance was a labor-sponsored and -financed organization that studied and proposed legislation on health insurance matters with special reference to national health insurance. It received major support from the United Automobile Workers, had developed a Washington "presence," and was viewed as an able and responsible voice for universal coverage.

31. For Rube Goldberg "inventions" and the significance of this reference, see *www.rube-goldberg.com/html/gallery.htm*.

32. Statement by Secretary Patricia Roberts Harris before a joint session of the House Ways and Means Committee and House Commerce Committee, Nov. 29, 1979, in *National Health Insurance: Working Papers*, vol. 2, p. 20.

33. Julius B. Richmond and Rashi Fein, "The Health Care Mess: A Bit of History," *JAMA* 273, No. 1 (1995), pp. 69–71.

34. For an account of the impact of Medicare on the hospital sector, see Rosemary Stevens, *In Sickness and in Wealth: American Hospitals in the Twentieth Century* (Baltimore: Johns Hopkins University Press, 1998).

35. Steffie Woolhandler and David U. Himmelstein, "When Money Is the Mission—The High Costs of Investor-Owned Care," *NEJM* 341, No. 6 (1999), pp. 444–446.

36. John B. McKinlay and John D. Stoeckle, "Corporatization and the Social Transformation of Doctoring," *International Journal of Health Services* 18 (1988), pp. 191–205.

37. Eli Ginzberg, "Monetarization of Medical Care," *NEJM* 310, No. 18 (1984), pp. 1162–1165.

38. Arnold S. Relman, "The Future of Medical Practice," *Health Affairs* 2, No. 2 (1983), pp. 5–19.

4. Education for the Health Professions

1. Bernard Guyer, Mary Ann Freedman, Donna M. Strobino, and Edward J. Sondik, "Annual Summary of Vital Statistics: Trends in the Health of Americans during the 20th Century," *Pediatrics* 106, No. 6 (2000), pp. 1307–1317; National Center for Health Statistics, "Deaths: Final Data for 2000," *National Vital Statistics Report* 50, No. 15 (2002), p. 1, at *http://www.cdc.gov/nchs/nvsr/nvsr50/nvsr50_15.pdf*.

2. United States Census Bureau, "The 65 Years and Over Population: 2000—Census 2000 Brief," Publication No. C2KBR/01-10 (October 2001), at *http://www.census.gov/prod/2001pubs/c2kbr01-10.pdf*.

3. Population data from United States Bureau of the Census, "Table DP-1—Profile of General Demographic Characteristics for the United States: 2000," *Census 2000*, at *http://www.census.gov/Press-Release/www/2001/rables/dp_us-2000.pdf*. Death rates from National Center for Health Statistics, *Health, United States, 2003* (Hyattsville, Md.: NCHS, 2003).

4. See *www.cdc.gov/nchs/faststats/infmort.htm*.

5. John P. Bunker, Howard S. Frazier, and Frederick Mosteller, "Improving Health: Measuring Effects of Medical Care," *The Milbank Quarterly* 72, No. 2

(1994), pp. 225–258. Thomas McKeown has written extensively on this matter. See, for example, McKeown, *The Role of Medicine: Dream, Mirage, or Nemesis?* 2d ed. (Princeton: Princeton University Press, 1979).

6. United States Department of Health, Education, and Welfare (HEW), *Healthy People: The Surgeon General's Report on Health Promotion and Disease Prevention*, Publication No. (PHS) 79-55071 (Washington: U.S. Government Printing Office, 1979).

7. United States Department of Health and Human Services, *Promoting Health, Preventing Disease: Objectives for the Nation* (Washington: U.S. Government Printing Office, 1980).

8. United States Department of Health and Human Services, *Healthy People 2000: National Health Promotion and Disease Prevention Objectives*, Publication No. (PHS) 91-50213 (Washington: U.S. Public Health Service, 1990); *Healthy People 2010, 2nd ed., with Understanding and Improving Health and Objectives for Improving Health*, 2 vols. (Washington: U.S. Government Printing Office, 2000).

9. See *www.hsps.org/userfiles/2003ADR.pdf*. An additional three schools were added in 2004.

10. Allan M. Brandt and Martha Gardner, "Antagonism and Accommodation: Interpreting the Relationship between Public Health and Medicine in the United States during the 20th Century," *American Journal of Public Health* 90, No. 5 (2000), pp. 707–715.

11. United States Department of Health, Education, and Welfare, *Smoking and Health: Report of the Advisory Committee to the Surgeon General of the Public Health Service*, Public Health Service Publication No. 1103 (Washington: U.S. Government Printing Office, 1964).

12. For example, in 1978 the tobacco industry spent $2 billion annually for the promotion of smoking. In contrast, because of the constraints imposed by members of Congress from tobacco-growing districts, the United States Public Health Service received $10 million (one-half of one percent of industry's expenditures) for its educational efforts.

13. American Cancer Society, *Cancer Facts and Figures 2001* (Atlanta: American Cancer Society, 2001), p. 29; Omar Shafey, Suzanne Dolwick, and G. Emmanuel Guindon, eds., *Tobacco Control Country Profiles 2003* (Atlanta: American Cancer Society, 2003), pp. 418–419. Available at *http://www.who.int/tobacco/global_data/country_profiles/en/* or at *http://www.globalink.org/tccp*.

14. The early history of the NIH is presented in Victoria Harden's *Inventing the NIH: Federal Biomedical Research Policy 1887–1937* (Baltimore: Johns Hopkins University Press, 1986). See also Stephen P. Strickland, *Story of the NIH Grants Program* (Lanham, Md.: Rowman and Littlefield, 1969, 1989).

15. Appropriations reached $11 billion in 1995, and then because of a congressional "commitment" to even more rapid growth, to almost $18 billion in

2000, and $27 billion in 2003. The NIH Almanac—Appropriations, *http://www .nih.gov.*

16. Clark Kerr, *The Uses of the University* (Cambridge, Mass.: Harvard University Press, 1963); Derek Bok, *Universities in the Market Place: The Commercialization of Higher Education* (Princeton: Princeton University Press, 2003).

17. David E. Rogers, "Reflections on a Medical School Deanship," *Pharos of Alpha Omega Alpha* 38, No. 3 (1975), pp. 115–121.

18. The term was still used in some medical centers years later about all patients.

19. Carnegie Commission on Higher Education, *Higher Education and the Nation's Health: Policies for Medical and Dental Education—A Special Report and Recommendations* (New York: McGraw-Hill, 1970).

20. Eli Ginzberg, ed., *Regionalization and Health Policy,* HEW Publication No. (HRA) 77-623 (Washington: U.S. Government Printing Office, 1977), pp. 107–119.

21. Julius B. Richmond, *Currents in American Medicine: A Developmental View of Medical Care and Medical Education* (Cambridge, Mass.: Harvard University Press, 1969), p. 45.

22. During the war students completed their program in three years by eliminating vacation periods.

23. Richmond, *Currents in American Medicine,* p. 6.

24. Ibid., pp. 6–7; Bureau of Health Professions, "Third Report to the President and Congress on the Status of Health Professions Personnel in the United States," HSS Publication No. (HRA) 82-2 (Hyattsville, Md.: Health Resources Administration, 1982).

25. United States Department of Health, Education, and Welfare, *A Report to the President on Medical Care Prices* (Washington: U.S. Government Printing Office, 1967).

26. Physicians for a Growing America, *Report of the Surgeon General's Consultant Group on Medical Education* (Washington: U.S. Government Printing Office, 1959).

27. Rashi Fein, *The Doctor Shortage: An Economic Diagnosis* (Washington: Brookings Institution, 1967).

28. During his tenure as Assistant Secretary for Health (1969–1971), Dr. Roger Egeberg, former dean of the medical school at the University of Southern California, would use the following artful phrasing in public speeches: "people tell me that we need 50,000 additional doctors." He thus avoided the problem of justifying the numbers. Dr. Fein recalls asking a group of medical leaders the basis for the statement that America needed 40,000 more physicians. He was told that whatever the number America had, it needed 40,000 more.

29. An excellent review of physician supply is found in David Blumenthal, "New Steam from an Old Cauldron: The Physician Supply Debate," *NEJM* 350 (2004), pp. 1780–1787.

30. Eric Redman, *Dance of Legislation* (New York: Simon & Schuster, 1973).

31. This discriminatory behavior was often rationalized with the observation that because of child-bearing and family needs, women would not practice as much as men, and that, given the need for physicians, it would be irresponsible to use (that is, "waste") scarce medical school slots to train persons who would not provide as many hours of care over their lifetimes. There was little evidence that this view had empirical justification; however, there was much evidence that medical schools and their teaching hospitals were unwilling to make any changes that would increase opportunities and facilitate greater participation by women.

32. Graduate Medical Education National Advisory Committee, *Report of the Graduate Medical Education National Advisory Committee to the Secretary, Department of Health and Human Services,* HHS Publication No. (HRA) 81-651 (Washington: U.S. Government Printing Office, 1980).

33. American Medical Association, *U.S. Medical Licensure Statistics 1985 and Licensure Requirements 1986* (Chicago: AMA Division of Survey and Data Resources, 1986), Tables 4 and 5.

34. As noted above, in an earlier time a space argument had been invoked to bar women from medical school. One applicant, who went on to a most distinguished career in medicine, public health, and government service at the local and federal level, was rejected by an Ivy League medical school on the grounds that she would have had to dissect a cadaver in the presence of males, that this was unacceptable, and that the cadaver could not be transported to a more "private" location.

35. There were occasional suggestions that producing an oversupply of physicians would create competition and thereby reduce fees and individual physician incomes. In turn, this might stimulate the growth of HMOs as physicians looked for assured employment. This view never gained wide acceptance.

36. Richmond, *Currents in American Medicine,* p. 38.

37. Ibid., p. 117.

38. George E. Miller, *Teaching and Learning in Medical School* (Cambridge, Mass.: Harvard University Press, 1961); George E. Miller and Fulap Tamas, eds., *Educational Strategies for Health Professions* (Geneva: World Health Organization, 1974); George E. Miller, *Educating Medical Teachers* (Cambridge, Mass.: Harvard University Press, 1980); Kenneth M. Ludmerer, *Time to Heal* (New York: Oxford University Press, 1999).

39. Institute of Medicine, Division of Health Sciences Policy, *Medical Education and Societal Needs: A Planning Report for Health Professions* (Washington:

National Academy Press, 1983), at *http://www.nap.edu/books/POD079/html/203 .html.*

40. Rashi Fein and Gerald I. Weber, *Financing Medical Education: An Analysis of Alternative Policies and Mechanisms* (New York: McGraw-Hill, 1971).

41. Richmond, *Currents in American Medicine*, pp. 113–123.

42. George L. Engel, "Sounding Board: The Biopsychosocial Model and Medical Education—'Who Are to Be the Teachers?'" *NEJM* 306, No. 13 (1982), pp. 802–805.

43. Lynn Haslett, "1969: McMaster University Introduces Problem-based Learning in Medical Education," in Daniel Schugurensky, ed., *History of Education: Selected Moments of the 20th Century* (2001), at *http://fcis.oise.utoronto.ca/~daniel_schugurensky/assignment1/1969mcmaster.html.*

44. Daniel C. Tosteson et al., *New Pathway to Medical Education: Learning to Learn at Harvard Medical School* (Cambridge, Mass.: Harvard University Press, 1994).

45. There is a rich literature on the subject of specialty selection. The annual education issue of the *Journal of the American Medical Association,* appearing in September, has much information. See especially Volume 292, No. 9 (2004). See also James Thornton, "Physician Choice of Medical Specialty: Do Economic Incentives Matter?" in *Applied Economics* 32, No. 11 (2000), pp. 1419–1428, and Nancy Stillwell, "Myers-Briggs Type and Medical Specialty Choice: A New Look at an Old Question," in *Teaching and Learning in Medicine* 12, No. 1 (2000), pp. 14–20.

46. See Ruth-Marie E. Fincher, "The Road Less Traveled—Attracting Students to Primary Care," *NEJM* 351, No. 7 (2004), pp. 630–632, and Michael E. Whitcomb and Jordan J. Cohen, "The Future of Primary Care Medicine," *NEJM* 351, No. 7 (2004), pp. 710–712.

47. See the pioneering studies by Wennberg on geographic variations in patterns of practice, such as John E. Wennberg and M. M. Cooper, eds., *The Quality of Medical Care in the United States: A Report on the Medicare Program—The Dartmouth Atlas of Health Care 1999* (Chicago: American Hospital Association Press, 1999).

48. John E. Wennberg, "Dealing with Medical Practice Variations: A Proposal for Action," *Health Affairs* 3, No. 2 (1984), pp. 6–32; John E. Wennberg, Eliot S. Fisher, and J. S. Skinner, "Geography and the Debate over Medicare Reform," *Health Affairs,* supplemental Web exclusives (Feb. 13, 2002), W96–114. Available at *http://content.healthaffairs.org/cgi/reprint/hlthaff.w2.96v1.*

49. Kurt Eichenwald, "Operating Profits: Mining Medicare—How One Hospital Benefited from Questionable Surgery," *New York Times* (April 12, 2003), p. A1.

50. Marcia Angell, "Is Academic Medicine for Sale?" *NEJM* 342, No. 20

(2000), pp. 1516–1518. See also Marcia Angell, *The Truth about Drug Companies: How They Deceive Us and What to Do about It* (New York: Random House, 2004); Jerome P. Kassirer, *On the Take: How Medicine's Complicity with Big Business Can Endanger Your Health* (New York: Oxford University Press, 2004); Jerry Avorn, *Powerful Medicines: The Benefits, Risks, and Costs of Prescription Drugs* (New York: Knopf, 2004).

51. See Earl P. Steinberg, "Improving the Quality of Care—Can We Practice What We Preach?" *NEJM* 348, No. 26 (June 26, 2003), pp. 2681–2683.

5. The Entrepreneurial Revolution

1. Between 1970 and 1995 approximately 7 percent (330 of approximately 5,000 private not-for-profit general medical and surgical hospitals) had converted to for-profit status. See David Cutler and Jill Horowitz, "Converting Hospitals from Not-for-Profit to For-Profit Status: Why and What Effects?" *National Bureau of Economic Research,* Working Paper No. 6672 (August 1998).

2. Medicaid is one of the sources of funding for long-term care. It is often the case that even if individuals enter the long-term care facility with private resources, these are used up over a period of time. The individual who has "spent down" may then qualify for Medicaid assistance.

3. Julius B. Richmond, *Currents in American Medicine: A Developmental View of Medical Care and Education* (Cambridge, Mass.: Harvard University Press, 1969), pp. 9, 22–24.

4. Ibid., pp. 9–11. See also Sam Zeller, "Lobbying: Identity Crisis," *National Journal* (April 27, 2002).

5. Kate Mulligan, "AMA Wrestles with Future—Medicare's and Its Own," *Psychiatric News* 38, No. 2 (2003), p. 1, at *http://pn.psychiatryonline.org/cgi/content/full/38/2/1.*

6. David B. Larson, Maria Chandler, and Howard P. Forman, "MD/MBA Programs in the United States: Evidence of a Change in Health Care Leadership," *Academic Medicine* 78, No. 3 (2003), pp. 335–341.

7. Rashi Fein, "What Is Wrong with the Language of Medicine?" *NEJM* 306, No. 14 (1982), pp. 863–864.

8. Jerome P. Kassirer, "Medicine at Center Stage," *NEJM* 328, No. 14 (1993), p. 1268.

9. John D. Stoeckle, "Reflections on Modern Doctoring," *The Milbank Quarterly* 66 (1988), pp. 76–91; John McKinlay and Joan Archer, "Towards the Proletarianization of Physicians," *International Journal of Health Services* 15 (1985), pp. 161–195; John McKinlay and John D. Stoeckle, "Corporatization and the Social Transformation of Doctoring," *International Journal of Health Services* 18 (1988), pp. 191–205.

10. Andrew C. Yacht, "Collective Bargaining Is the Right Step," *NEJM* 342, No. 6 (2000), pp. 429–431; American College of Physicians, American Society of Internal Medicine, "Physicians and Joint Negotiations: A Position Paper," *Annals of Internal Medicine* 134, No. 9 (2001), pp. 787–792.

11. Eli Ginzberg, "The Destabilization of Health Care," *NEJM* 315, No. 12 (1986), pp. 757–761.

12. Steffie Woolhandler and David U. Himmelstein, "Extreme Risk: The New Corporate Proposition for Physicians," *NEJM* 333, No. 25 (1995), pp. 1706–1708.

13. Similar ethical issues may arise when physicians own (or have an economic interest in) diagnostic facilities and/or laboratories.

14. Symmetry suggests (and the facts bear out) that insurance companies entered the field of managed care and tried to organize delivery systems without adequate understanding of what it took to run an organization that intersected with patients in a manner quite different from mailing a bill, collecting a premium, paying providers, and calculating risks.

15. David U. Himmelstein and Steffie Woolhandler, "Bound to Gag," *Archives of Internal Medicine* 157, No. 18 (1997), p. 2033.

16. Dr. Fein recalls that when his physician suggested that it no longer was necessary to have an ultrasound examination annually and that it would be sufficient to have the examination every three to five years, he had to assure his daughter that judgment reflected the physician's standard of care, not HMO pressure.

17. *John Q.* (2002) is the story of a blue-collar family whose health insurance proves insufficient to cover the emergency heart transplant needed to save their young son. Unable to raise sufficient funds, and unwilling to bring the son home to die, the father takes members of the hospital staff hostage, promising to release them after the needed operation for his son. See also Elizabeth A. Pendo, "Images of Health Insurance in Popular Film: The Dissolving Critique," *Journal of Health Law* 37 (Spring 2004), pp. 267–315, at *http://ssrn.com/abstract=578321.*

18. John K. Iglehart, "Medicaid Turns to Prepaid Managed Care," *NEJM* 308, No. 16 (1983), pp. 976–980.

19. On June 21, 2004, a unanimous United States Supreme Court ruled that the Employee Retirement Income Security Act (ERISA) of 1974 (the federal law that governs employer-based benefit plans) preempted claims filed in state courts against HMOs for failing to pay for care that had been recommended by an HMO physician. This removed punitive damages and other state law remedies, and limited claims against the HMO to those that could be filed under ERISA (largely the monetary value of the benefit). Justice Ruth Bader Ginsburg bemoaned the lack of recourse available to patients, and suggested

that Congress amend ERISA in order to provide for a complete remedy option. See *www.cga.state.ct.us/2004/rpt/2004-R-0550.htm.*

20. Robert Pear, "Spending on Health Care Increased Sharply in 2001," *New York Times* (Jan. 8, 2003), p. A12; Katharine Levit, Cynthia Smith, Cathy Cowan, Art Sensenig, Aaron Catlin, and the Health Accounts Team, "Health Spending Rebound Continues in 2002," *Health Affairs* 23, No. 1 (2004), pp. 147–159.

21. National Center for Health Statistics, *Health, United States, 2003: With Chartbook on Trends in the Health of Americans* (Hyattsville, Md.: 2002), p. 307, Table 113.

22. Grantmakers in Health is a nonprofit group that tracks the emergence and activities of all health foundations. Its report, *A Profile of New Health Foundations, May 2003,* includes basic information about 153 of the 165 health foundations that currently exist. The cumulative assets of these foundations now reach $16.4 billion, with a median asset value of $46.5 million. Over 59 percent of these foundations were formed between 1994 and 1999, and an additional 11 percent since 1999. See *http://www.gih.org/usr_doc/2003_Profile_Report .pdf.*

23. The *New York Times* headlined a survey of magnetic resonance imaging (MRI) machines: Reed Abelson, "An M.R.I. Machine for Every Doctor? Someone Has to Pay," *New York Times* (March 13, 2004), p. A1.

24. "Health Care Reform and the 1992 Presidential Election," *Kaiser Health Poll Report* (January–February 2004).

25. Robin Toner, "Washington at Work; The Clintons' Health Care Nemesis: The Man behind 'Harry and Louise,'" *New York Times* (April 6, 1994), p. A18.

26. For additional perspectives on the Clinton health program failure, see Haynes Johnson and David Broder, *The System: The American Way of Politics at the Breaking Point* (New York: Little, Brown and Co., 1996), and Theda Skocpol, *Boomerang: Health Care Reform and the Turn against Government* (New York: W. W. Norton, 1997).

27. Robert J. Blendon, Mollyann Brodie, and John M. Benson, "What Happened to Americans' Support for the Clinton Plan?" *Health Affairs* 14, No. 2 (1995), pp. 7–23.

28. Elinor Langer, "Who Makes Our Health Policy?" *Physicians' Forum* (June 1967), p. 5.

29. Robert J. Blendon and John M. Benson, "Americans' Views on Health Policy: A Fifty-Year Historical Perspective," *Health Affairs* 20, No. 2 (2001), pp. 33–46.

30. United States Census Bureau, *Statistical Abstract of the United States: 1999* (Washington: U.S. Department of Commerce, Economics and Statistics Administration, Bureau of the Census, 2000), p. 127, Table 185.

31. See *http://www.cobrainsurance.com/COBRA_Law.htm*.

32. See *http://cms.hhs.gov/hipaa*.

33. Centers for Medicare and Medicaid Services, "FY 2003: Number of Children Ever Enrolled in SCHIP by Program Type," at *http://www.com.hhs.gov/schip/enrollment/schip03.pdf*.

34. For the Women's Health and Cancer Rights Act (WHCRA) of 1998, see *http://www.cms.hhs.gov/hipaa/hipaa1/content/whcra.asp*; for the Mental Health Parity Act (MHPA) of 1996, see *http://www.cms.hhs.gov/hipaa/hipaa1/content/mhpa.asp*; for the Newborns' and Mothers' Health Protection Act (NMHPA) of 1996, see *http://www.cms.hhs.gov/hipaa/hipaa1/content/nmhpa.asp*.

35. AcademyHealth considers itself the "professional home for health service researchers, policy analysts, and practitioners, and a leading non-partisan source for the best in health research and policy." See *http://academyhealth.org/about/index.htm*.

36. Archibald L. Cochrane, *Effectiveness and Efficiency: Random Reflections on the Health Services* (London: Nuffield Provincial Hospitals Trust, 1972).

37. *Smoking and Health: Report of the Advisory Committee to the Surgeon General of the Public Health Service* (Washington: U.S. Department of Health, Education, and Welfare, Public Health Service, 1964).

38. Institute of Medicine, Committee on Quality of Health in America, *To Err Is Human: Building a Better Health System* (Washington: National Academy Press, 1999).

39. Institute of Medicine, Committee on Quality of Health in America, *Crossing the Quality Chasm: A New Health System for the 21st Century* (Washington: National Academy Press, 2001).

40. See the work of Donald Berwick and of the Institute for Healthcare Improvement, which he heads. The institute is a "non-profit organization dedicated to improving the quality of health care systems through education, research, and demonstration projects, and through fostering collaboration among health care organizations and their leaders."

41. Nevertheless, computers may also facilitate prescription error risks. See Ross Koppel et al., "Role of Computerized Physician Order Entry Systems in Facilitating Medication Errors," *JAMA* 293, No. 10 (2005), pp. 1197–1203.

42. According to its official website, the AHRQ, which replaced the Agency for Health Care Policy and Research in 1999, as "a part of the U.S. Department of Health and Human Services, is the lead agency charged with supporting research designed to improve the quality of healthcare, reduce its cost, improve patient safety, decrease medical errors, and broaden access to essential services. AHRQ sponsors and conducts research that provides evidence-based information on healthcare outcomes; quality; and cost, use, and access." See *http://www.ahcpr.gov/about/ahrqfact.htm*.

43. J. P. Newhouse et al., "Some Interim Results from a Controlled Trial of Cost Sharing in Health Insurance," *NEJM* 305, No. 25 (1981), pp. 1501–1507.

44. Robert Pear, "Fewer People on Medicare Dropped by HMOs," *New York Times* (Sept. 9, 2003), p. A27.

45. Fred Charatan, "Health Maintenance Organisations Drop Medicare Beneficiaries," *British Medical Journal* 323, No. 7316 (2001), p. 772.

46. Steffie Woolhandler, David U. Himmelstein, and James P. Lewontin, "Administrative Costs in US Hospitals," *NEJM* 329, No. 6 (1993), pp. 400–403; Steffie Woolhandler and David U. Himmelstein, "Cost of Care and Administration at For-Profit and Other Hospitals in the United States," *NEJM* 336, No. 11 (1997), pp. 769–774.

47. Barbara Whitaker, "Changing of the Managed-Care Guard," *New York Times* (Nov. 28, 1999), sec. 3, p. 11.

6. Beyond the Dollars

1. John P. Bunker, Howard S. Frazier, and Frederick Mosteller, "Improving Health: Measuring Effects of Medical Care," *The Milbank Quarterly* 72, No. 2 (1994), pp. 225–258.

2. Some therapeutic advances, such as the treatment of childhood acute leukemia and of Hodgkin's disease, were remarkably effective. These improvements, however, did not have a major impact on vital statistics because of the relatively small numbers of patients.

3. Julius B. Richmond, *Currents in American Medicine: A Developmental View of Medical Care and Medical Education* (Cambridge, Mass.: Harvard University Press, 1969), pp. 94–95.

4. Institute of Medicine, Committee on the NIH Research Priority-Setting Process, *Scientific Opportunities and Public Needs: Improving Priority Setting and Public Input at NIH* (Washington: National Academy Press, 1998).

5. Christine Bahls, "NIH Budget Tracks Doubling Goal," *Scientist* 15, No. 22 (2001), p. 10.

6. John G. Freymaun, "The Origins of Disease Orientation in American Medical Education," *Preventive Medicine* 10 (1981), pp. 663–673.

7. Thomas Parran, *Shadow on the Land: Syphilis* (New York: Reynal and Hitchcock, 1937).

8. In 1988 the then-Surgeon-General, Dr. C. Everett Koop, sent a brochure entitled "Understanding AIDS" to each of the 107 million households in the United States, becoming the largest mailing on public health in American history.

9. L. Lasker, "Is There a Better Way to Secure Funding for Medical Re-

search?" *Scientist* 10, No. 2 (1996), p. 10; Stephen P. Strickland, *The Story of the NIH Grants Programs* (Lanham, Md.: University Press of America, 1989).

10. Jo Ivey Boufford and Phillip R. Lee, *Health Policies for the 21st Century: Challenges and Recommendations for the U.S. Department of Health and Human Services* (New York: Milbank Memorial Fund, 2001), p. 2.

11. Katharine Levit, Cynthia Smith, Cathy Cowan, Art Sensenig, Aaron Catlin, and the Health Accounts Team, "Health Spending Rebound Continues in 2002," *Health Affairs* 23, No. 1 (2004), pp. 147–159.

12. "FY 2003 President's Budget for HHS," at *http://www.hhs.gov/budget/docbudget.htm.*

13. Social Security Act §1801 (42 U.S.C. 1395), at *http://www.ssa.gov/op_home/ssact/title18/1800.htm.*

14. Edward D. Berkowitz, *To Improve Human Health: A History of the Institute of Medicine* (Washington: National Academy Press, 1998).

15. Institute of Medicine, Committee for the Study of the Future of Public Health, *The Future of Public Health* (Washington: National Academy Press, 1988).

16. Anthony S. Fauci, "Smallpox Vaccination Policy: The Need for Dialogue," *NEJM* 346, No. 17 (2002), pp. 1319–1320.

17. *Quantitative Skills:* Epidemiology and biostatistics were considered core disciplines, and all students needed to acquire the basic quantitative skills required to evaluate or conduct population-based studies. *Health of Populations:* This emphasis led to an interest in the public policies of agencies such as the Environmental Protection Agency, the Occupational Safety and Health Administration, the Centers for Disease Control, and the Food and Drug Administration. Organized labor and many consumer and voluntary health organizations stimulated studies in schools of public health. The appearance of HIV infections and AIDS in the 1980s renewed interest in and concern with population-based infectious disease research. *Management and Finance:* Research and training programs in this field evolved as the health sector kept growing in expenditures and complexity. Given the need for managers of health care programs and institutions as well as for public health efforts, this area of training received much attention. *International Health Issues:* The health problems of developing countries, many of which had not yet gone through the transition to infectious disease control, received considerable focus. Many students came from those countries, and international health organizations and agencies often collaborated with schools of public health in arranging training programs. The role of these entities in worldwide efforts to improve health was taught to all students, and exchange programs were fostered to help American students learn more about international health. See Allan Brandt and Martha

Gardner, "Antagonism and Accommodation: Interpreting the Relationship between Public Health and Medicine in the United States during the 20th Century," *American Journal of Public Health* 90, No. 5 (2000), pp. 707–715. Also see Institute of Medicine, Committee on Public Health, *Healthy Communities: New Partnerships for the Future of Public Health* (Washington: National Academy Press, 1996).

18. Richmond, *Currents in American Medicine*, Chapter 2.

19. Ibid., p. 28.

20. David Nathan, "Clinical Research: Perceptions, Reality, and Proposed Solutions," *JAMA* 280, No. 16 (1998), pp. 1427–1431. Nathan comments on and gives background to the report of the NIH director's panel on clinical research. The final report (1997) is available at *http://www.nih.gov/news/crp/97report/execsum.htm*.

21. These are all discussed more fully in the next chapter.

22. Derek Bok, *Universities in the Marketplace: The Commercialization of Higher Education* (Princeton, N.J.: Princeton University Press, 2003); see also *http://www.warf.ws/aboutus/index.jsp?catid=39*. See Donald Kennedy, "Editorial, Bayh-Dole: Almost 25," *Science* 307, No. 5714 (2005), p. 1375.

23. "Uniform Requirements of the International Committee of Journal Editors," at *www.ICMJF.org* (2003).

24. The *New York Times* (July 20, 2004), p. F7, reports that NIH "acknowledged that eight of nine experts on the panel that issued the recommendations [concerning sharply lowering desired levels of harmful cholesterol and the use of statins] had received financing from one or more of the companies that make statins." Dr. James Cleeland, coordinator of the National Cholesterol Education Program, stated that "if you excluded all the people who have any financial connection to industry, you'd exclude all the people who are most expert."

25. Marcia Angell, "Is Academic Medicine for Sale?" *NEJM* 342, No. 20 (2000), pp. 1516–1518; AAMC, Task Force on Financial Conflicts of Interest in Clinical Research, *Protecting Subjects, Preserving Trust, Promoting Progress: Policy and Guidelines for the Oversight of Individual Financial Interests in Human Subjects Research* (Washington: AAMC, 2001); AAMC, *Protecting Subjects, Preserving Trust, Promoting Progress II: Principles and Recommendations for Oversight of an Institution's Financial Interests in Human Subjects Research* (Washington: AAMC, 2002); Hamilton Moses III, Eugene Braunwald, Joseph B. Martin, and Samuel O. Thier, "Collaborating with Industry—Choices for the Academic Health Center," *NEJM* 347, No. 17 (2002), pp. 1371–1375; Jocelyn Kaiser, "Proposed Rules Aim to Curb Financial Conflicts of Interest," *Science* 295, No. 5553 (2002), pp. 246–247.

26. Arnold S. Relman and Marcia Angell, "America's Other Drug Problem: How the Drug Industry Distorts Medicine and Politics," *New Republic* 227, No.

25 (Dec. 16, 2002), pp. 27–41.

27. David Stout, "Drug Makers Get Leeway on TV Ads," *New York Times* (Aug. 9, 1997), sec. 1, p. 35.

28. Allan Brandt, *No Magic Bullet: A Social History of Venereal Disease in the United States since 1880* (New York: Oxford University Press, 1987).

29. See Advisory Committee on Human Radiation Experiments, *The Human Radiation Experiments* (New York: Oxford University Press, 1996).

30. National Institutes of Health, Office for Human Research Protection, "Code of Federal Regulations: Title 45 Public Welfare, Part 46 Protection of Human Subjects," revised Nov. 13, 2001. See *http://ohrp.osophs.dhhs.gov/human subjects/guidance/45cfr46.htm.*

31. See, for example, Peter G. Gosselin, "Congress to Probe Conduct in Clinical Tests," *Boston Globe* (Oct. 20, 1988), National/Foreign section, p. 1; "Fraud Inquiry Aims at AIDS Researcher," *St. Louis Post-Dispatch* (July 16, 1989), p. 1A; Phillip J. Hilts, "How Investigation of Lab Fraud Grew into a Cause Celebre," *New York Times* (March 16, 1991), p. C1.

32. For a concise history of the Office of Research Integrity, visit *http:// ori.dhhs.gov/html/about/historical.asp.* For a concise history of the Office of Human Research Protections, see *http://www.hhs.gov/news/press/2000pres/20000 606a.html.*

33. Lisa Lehmann et al., "A Survey of Medical Ethics Education at the U.S. and Canadian Medical Schools," *Academic Medicine* 79 (2004), pp. 682–689.

34. A list of the various Presidential commissions that examined ethical issues can be found at *http://www.bioethics.gov/reports/past_commissions.*

35. Richmond, *Currents in American Medicine,* p. 125, n. 22.

36. The Association of American Medical Colleges publishes a monthly scholarly journal, *Academic Medicine,* which, according to its website, "serves as an international forum for the exchange of ideas and information on policy issues and research concerning academic medicine, including strengthening the quality of medical education and training, integrating education and research into the provision of effective health care, enhancing the search for biomedical knowledge, and advancing research in health sciences." See *http:// www .academicmedicine.org/misc/about.shtml.*

37. When the section was dropped in the spring of 2004, *JAMA* made clear that it did not view this as a retreat from its commitment to student interests. It stated that it was expanding student opportunity to publish and would provide resources to assist student authors in bringing this possibility to fruition.

38. Institute of Medicine, Committee on Quality of Health in America, *To Err Is Human: Building a Better Health System* (Washington: National Academy Press, 1999).

39. See *http://www.aamc.org/newsroom/reporter/sept03/exam.htm* for a full discussion of this new Step 2 Clinical Skills examination as a component of the

United States Medical Licensing Exam. The date of the examination was set by the National Board of Medical Examiners.

40. See Edward M. Hundert et al., "Characteristics of the Informal Curriculum and Trainees' Ethical Choices," *Academic Medicine* 71 (1996), pp. 624–642.

41. See *http://www.medschool.ucsf.edu/academy* and *http://academy.med.harvard.edu*.

42. Kenneth M. Ludmerer, *Time to Heal: American Medical Education from the Turn of the Century to the Era of Managed Care* (New York: Oxford University Press, 1999).

43. Janet A. Tighe, Review of "Iconoclast: Abraham Flexner and a Life in Learning," *JAMA* 289, No. 16 (2003), pp. 2147–2148.

44. Nicholas A. Christakis, "The Similarity and Frequency of Proposals to Reform US Medical Education: Constant Concerns," *JAMA* 274, No. 9 (1995), pp. 706–711.

45. Report of the Committee of Deans, "Educating Doctors to Provide High Quality Medical Care—A Vision for Medical Education in the United States," Association of American Medical Colleges (Washington, July 2004).

46. Amy C. Brodkey, Frederick S. Sierles, Ilyse L. Spertus, Cindy L. Weiner, and Fredrick A. McCurdy, "Clerkship Directors' Perceptions of the Effects of Managed Care on Medical Students' Education," *Academic Medicine* 77, No. 11 (2002), pp. 1112–1120.

47. Donald Nutter and Michael Whitcomb, *The AAMC Project on the Clinical Education of Medical Students,* Association of American Medical Colleges (Washington, 2004).

48. The 1997 Balanced Budget Act reduced the funds that teaching hospitals were to receive in subsequent years for indirect payments for medical education (IME) and set caps on the number of residents for whom there would be reimbursement for the direct costs of training for graduate medical education (GME). Both IME and GME funds come from Medicare Part A. IME payments have been significantly increased by the Medicare Prescription Drug, Improvement, and Modernization Act of 2003. See *http://www.aamc.org/advocacy/gme*.

49. That there are serious problems with the way medical education is financed is clear. Nevertheless, the problem of a shortage of clinicians able to free up the time to teach medical students clinical medicine could be solved with a relatively modest infusion of earmarked funds. A small surcharge on all health insurers is one way to raise the requisite sums.

50. "On July 2, 1862, President Abraham Lincoln signed into law what is generally referred to as the Land Grant Act. The new piece of legislation introduced by U.S. Representative Justin Smith Morrill of Vermont granted each state 30,000 acres of public land for each Senator and Representative under ap-

portionment based on the 1860 census. Proceeds from the sale of these lands were to be invested in a perpetual endowment fund which would provide support for colleges of agriculture and mechanical arts in each of the states." See *http://www.higher-ed.org/resources/morrill_acts.htm*. A list of institutions founded by this Act can be found at *http://www.higher-ed.org/resources/land_grant_colleges.htm*.

51. Between 1978 and 1981 nearly 6,700 scholarships were awarded. In 1987 Congress authorized the National Health Service Corps (NHSC) Loan Repayment Program, which enables the recruitment of clinicians for immediate service to shortage areas. See *http://nhsc.bhpr.hrsa.gov/about/our/where.cfm*.

52. See *http://www.aamc.org/newsroom/pressrel/2004/040426.htm*.

53. Rashi Fein and Gerald I. Weber, *Financing Medical Education: An Analysis of Alternative Policies and Mechanisms* (Washington: Brookings Institution, 1971).

54. Corolla Eisenberg, "It Is Still a Privilege to Be a Doctor?" *NEJM* 314, No. 17 (1986), pp. 1113–1114; Abigail Zuger, "Dissatisfaction with Medical Practice," *NEJM* 350, No. 1 (Jan. 1, 2004), pp. 69–75.

55. Graduate Medical Education National Advisory Committee, *Report of the Graduate Medical Education National Advisory Committee to the Secretary, Department of Health and Human Services* (Washington: U.S. Department of Health and Human Services, 1981).

56. Richard A. Cooper, Thomas E. Getzen, Heather J. McKee, and Prakash Laud, "Economic and Demographic Trends Signal an Impending Physician Shortage," *Health Affairs* 21, No. 1 (2002), pp. 140–154.

57. Fitzhugh Mullan, Robert M. Politzer, and C. Howard Davis, "Medical Migration and the Physician Workforce: International Medical Graduates and American Medicine—Special Communications," *JAMA* 273, No. 19 (1995), pp. 1521–1527.

58. Linda H. Aiken, "Achieving an Interdisciplinary Workforce in Health Care," *NEJM* 348, No. 2 (2003), pp. 164–166.

59. The new center is the AAMC Center for Physician Workforce Studies. The significance of this effort is discussed in "A Word from the President: Tackling the Physician Supply Issue," at *http://www.aamc.org/newsroom/reporter/feb04/word.htm*.

7. Medical Challenges and Opportunities

1. World Health Organization, *Global Plan to Stop TB* (Geneva: WHO, 2002), at *www.stoptb.org*.

2. Over the years there have been three major federal commissions on mental illness. The first was the Joint Commission on Mental Illness and

Health with its final report published as *Action for Mental Health* (New York: Basic Books, 1961). President Carter issued an Executive Order establishing the "President's Commission on Mental Health" in 1977; its final report was released in 1978. President George W. Bush established the commission "Transforming Mental Health: The President's New Freedom Commission on Mental Health" by Executive Order in April 2002. See also Robert Desjarlais et al., *World Mental Health* (New York: Oxford University Press, 1996), and World Health Organization, *The World Health Report 2001—Mental Health* (Geneva: WHO, 2001).

3. Jack Shonkoff and Deborah A. Phillips, eds., *From Neurons to Neighborhoods: The Science of Early Childhood Development* (Washington: National Academy Press, 2000).

4. See *http://www.cdc.gov/nccdphp/dnpa/obesity.*

5. See *http://content.healthaffairs.org/cgi/content/abstract/23/2/199.*

6. See The International Genome Sequencing Consortium, "Initial Sequencing and Analysis of the Human Genome," *Nature* 409 (2001), pp. 860–921, and the special issue devoted to the completion of the Human Genome Project by Celera in *Science* 291, No. 5507 (2001).

7. Susan E. Waisbren et al., "Effects of Expanded Newborn Screening for Biochemical Genetic Disorders on Child Outcomes and Parental Stress," *JAMA* 290 (2003), pp. 2564–2572.

8. United Network for Organ Sharing, "Organ Donation and Transplantation," at *http://www.unos.org/WhoWeAre/history.asp.*

9. Presidential Proclamation 6158 (July 17, 1990), at *http://www.loc.gov/loc/brain/proclaim.html.*

10. See *http://www.sfn.org.*

11. Joseph B. Martin, "Molecular Basis of the Neurodegenerative Disorders," *NEJM* 340 (1999), pp. 1970–1980.

12. Shonkoff and Phillips, eds., *From Neurons to Neighborhoods.*

13. Institute of Medicine, *Health Literacy: A Prescription to End Confusion* (Washington: National Academy Press, 2004).

14. National Center for Health Statistics, *Health, United States, 2003* (Washington: U.S. Government Printing Office, 2003), pp. 121–122, Table 19.

15. Ibid., pp. 159–161, Table 36.

16. Peter B. Black et al., "Primary Care Physicians Who Treat Blacks and Whites," *NEJM* 351 (2004), pp. 575–584, and Arnold M. Epstein, "Health Care in America—Still Too Separate, Not Yet Equal," *NEJM* 351 (2004), pp. 603–605.

17. John E. Wennberg and M. M. Cooper, eds., *The Quality of Medical Care in*

the United States: A Report on the Medicare Program—The Dartmouth Atlas of Health Care 1999 (Chicago: American Hospital Association Press, 1999).

18. Robert J. Haggerty, K. V. Roghmann, and Ivan B. Pless, eds., *Child Health and the Community* (New York: John Wiley & Sons, 1975).

19. J. Robert Oppenheimer, "Tree of Knowledge," *Harper's* (October 1958), p. 55.

20. One maldistribution problem can be explained by the fact that, beginning in 1998, the number of graduates entering primary care specialties has declined each year (and especially so in family practice). Michael E. Whitcomb and Jordan J. Cohen, "The Future of Primary Care Medicine," *JAMA* 351 (2004), pp. 710–712.

21. See Albert Crenshaw, "New Law Hands Teaching Hospitals an Antitrust Shield," *Washington Post* (April 13, 2004), p. A2; "AAMC Responds to Residents' Lawsuit," at *http://www.aamc.org/newsroom/jungcomplaint/start.htm;* Katherine S. Mangan, "Medical Students' Lawsuit Thrown Out," *Chronicle of Higher Education* (Sept. 3, 2004), p. A28.

22. See, for example, Kenneth Ludmerer, *Time to Heal* (New York: Oxford University Press, 1999).

23. But see David Mechanic et al., "Are Patients' Office Visits Getting Shorter?" *NEJM* 344 (2001), pp. 198–204.

24. It would be useful to revisit the numerous recommendations and supporting materials that have been put forward to address student tuition costs, student loans, and the financial aspects of medical education. See Rashi Fein and Gerald Weber, *Financing Medical Education* (New York: McGraw Hill, 1971). This volume was part of the Carnegie Commission Series on American Higher Education.

25. The issue of claims against manufacturers of pharmaceuticals and medical devices is important, but not part of the subject of our discussion on physician frustration.

26. See *http://www.drugintel.com/news/a30113/medical_malpractice_crisis.htm.*

27. See *http://www.usatoday.com/news/nation/2004–06–13-med-malpractice_x .htm.*

28. "Medical Malpractice Insurance: Multiple Factors Have Contributed to Increased Premium Rates," Government Accounting Office: GAO-03-702, released July 28, 2003, at *http://www.gao.gov/attext/d03701.txt,* 39 pages. See also "Implications of Rising Premiums on Access to Health Care: Medical Malpractice and Access to Health Care," Government Accounting Office: GAO-03-836, at *http://www.gao.gov/atext/d03836.txt,* 41 pages.

29. An especially useful report is found in David M. Studdert, Michelle M.

Mello, and Troyen A. Brennan, "Health Policy Report: Medical Malpractice," *NEJM* 350 (2004), pp. 283–292. See also Sasha Polakow-Suransky, "Bad Medicine: Why Bush's Malpractice Policy Will Only Help Insurers," *The American Prospect* 14, No. 7 (2003), pp. 59–62; Joseph B. Treaster, "Malpractice Insurance: No Clear or Easy Answers," *New York Times* (March 5, 2003), p. C1; Jane Gordon, "Doctors Upset over Malpractice; Patients Are, Too," *New York Times* (March 23, 2003), sec. 14CN, p. 1.

30. See *http://www.drugintel.com/news/a30113/medical_malpractice_crisis.htm.*

31. Sally Trude, "So Much to Do, So Little Time: Physician Capacity Constraints, 1997–2001," Center for Studying Health Systems Change (Washington, May 2003). Mechanic et al., in "Are Patients' Office Visits Getting Shorter?" present a contrasting view.

32. This phenomenon may apply more frequently to certain specialties than to others where the relationship extends over a longer period of time (as, for example, may be the case with obstetrics).

33. Studdert et al., in "Health Policy Report: Medical Malpractice," cite various studies that suggest that a very low proportion of negligent injuries (under 10 percent and, perhaps, as low as 2 percent) result in claims.

34. See Richard Harris, *The Sacred Trust* (New York: New American Library, 1966).

35. See *http://management.bu.edu/research/ISIMS/presentations/Gourville.ppt.*

36. See *http://www.chiroweb.com/archives/17/04/09.htm.*

37. It first presented its single payer proposal in an article, "A National Health Program for the United States: A Physicians' Proposal," *NEJM* 320 (1989), pp. 102–108. Its most recent contribution was "Proposal of Physicians Working Group for Single-Payer National Health Insurance," *JAMA* 290, No. 6 (2003), pp. 798–805.

38. But see Donald J. Palmisano, David W. Emmors, and Gregory D. Wozniak, "Expanding Insurance Coverage through Tax Credits—Consumer Choice and Market Enticements: The AMA Proposal for Health Insurance Reform," *JAMA* 291, No. 18 (2004), pp. 2237–2242. It is not clear whether this will lead to the profession's active participation in debates about the uninsured.

39. Jeffrey Brainard, "Is the Boom in U.S. Spending on Science a Mixed Blessing?" *Chronicle of Higher Education* 46, No. 11 (Nov. 5, 1999), p. A35.

40. Daniel P. Greenberg, *Science, Money, and Politics* (Chicago: University of Chicago Press, 2001).

41. Robert Steinbrook, "Financial Conflicts of Interest and the NIH," *NEJM* 350 (2004), pp. 327–330.

42. See Derek Bok, *Universities in the Marketplace: The Commercialization of Higher Education* (Princeton: Princeton University Press, 2003), and Association

of American Medical Colleges, Task Force on Financial Conflicts of Interest in Clinical Research, *Protecting Subjects, Preserving Trust, and Promoting Progress: Policy and Guidelines for the Oversight of Individual Financial Interests in Research* (Washington: AAMC, 2001).

43. This division is not synonymous with outpatient and hospital care since many specialized services are provided in outpatient settings.

44. A helpful report on academic health centers can be found in Task Force on Academic Health Centers, "Envisioning the Future of Academic Health Centers: Final Report of the Commonwealth Fund Task Force on Academic Health Centers," Commonwealth Fund (New York: May 2003). See also the various in-depth interim reports of the Task Force.

45. The greater Pittsburgh area, for example, has 160 MRI scanners, more than all the machines in Canada. As a consequence Highmark (a not-for-profit insurer that dominates the market) has decided to pay for advanced imaging procedures that meet its defined quality standards. See Vanessa Fuhrmans, "Health Insurer to Target Scans for Cost Cuts," *Wall Street Journal* (Aug. 19, 2004), p. B1.

46. Rashi Fein, "Factors Influencing the Location of North Carolina General Practitioners: A Study in Physician Distribution" (Ph.D. diss., Johns Hopkins University, 1956).

47. The federal government is questioning whether these arrangements violate the Medicare legislation that bans extra fees. See Robert Pear, "U.S. Warns about Care Doctors Offer for Extra Fees," *New York Times* (April 13, 2004), p. A18.

8. Increasing Equity

1. The confusion concerning health care as a "right" is illustrated by a situation encountered by Dr. Richmond as the first director of the national Head Start program. Since health services were to be part of the program, Head Start set about having all enrolled children examined. The AMA, in its opposition to Medicare, had often stated that nobody in America need go without medical care. But once the Head Start program identified many children who required health care services, medical societies began to complain that they could not meet the newly documented need. They had to be reminded that the program had not generated the "need." All it had done was generate the demand.

2. We do not view the 2003 "expansion" of Medicare to cover pharmaceuticals (beginning in 2006) and to enable various Medicare and general insurance "reform" initiatives as significant steps forward. What is truly significant are individual medical savings accounts that provide greater tax relief

to upper-income groups and that are likely to fragment, if not destroy, the insurance market. What is likely to prove equally noteworthy about the legislation is the shift from traditional Medicare to a greater reliance on the private sector for insurance coverage, and the provision of subsidies to enterprises in the private sector to induce them to expand and provide such coverage for Medicare beneficiaries; the willingness to relate the premium for Part B Medicare to beneficiary income and other changes in traditional social insurance arrangements; and the demonstration of the power of the Pharmaceutical Manufacturers of America to advance its interests. In our judgment, the legislation will undergo substantive revision within a very few years after implementation. We believe that it is likely that many of the initiatives will be cut back.

3. Julius B. Richmond aphorism.

4. See *http://ferret.bls.census.gov/macro/032004/health/h01_001.htm.*

5. Comprehensive data and bibliographic references are available at *http:// www.covertheuninsuredweek.org/materials/files/IssuesGuide/pdf.*

6. For a full discussion of the methodology involved in these estimates, see Jack Hadley and John Holahan, "Covering the Uninsured: How Much Would It Cost?" *Health Affairs,* Web exclusives (January–June 2003).

7. Jack Hadley and John Holahan, "The Cost of Care for the Uninsured: What Do We Pay, Who Pays, and What Would Full Coverage Add to Medical Spending?" Kaiser Commission on Medicaid and the Uninsured (May 10, 2004), pp. 1–14, at *http://www.kff.org/universal/7084.cfm.*

8. Ibid., p. 5.

9. Ibid., p. 15.

10. Jack Hadley, "Sicker and Poorer—The Consequences of Being Uninsured," *Medical Care Research and Review* 60, No. 2 (June 2003).

11. Institute of Medicine, *Care without Coverage: Too Little, Too Late* (Washington: National Academy Press, 2002), pp. 161–165.

12. Institute of Medicine, *Hidden Costs, Value Lost* (Washington: National Academy Press, 2003), p. 112.

13. Even as not-for-profit hospitals used the term "profit," they decried Attorneys General who wanted to know more about their contributions to the community as not-for-profit entities. Some states attempted to impose taxes on hospitals that claimed not-for-profit status but, in the eyes of taxing authorities, behaved as for-profits.

14. This is the approach advocated by the Physicians for a National Health Plan, which rejects an incremental approach. See "Proposal of the Physicians' Working Group for Single-Payer National Health Insurance," *JAMA* 290

(2003), pp. 798–805, and Rashi Fein, "Universal Health Insurance: Let the Debate Resume," *JAMA* 290 (2003), pp. 818–820.

15. Barry Schwartz, "Nation of Second Guesses," *New York Times,* op-ed (Jan. 22, 2004). See also Barry Schwartz, *The Paradox of Choice: Why More Is Less* (New York: Ecco, 2004).

16. The term "single payer" seems to conflate three critical issues: that there be a single enrollment mechanism and organization, that there be a single collector of funds, and that there be a single payer of bills. At various times there have been suggestions for single payer mechanisms that relied on multiple enrollments. The latter proposals do not embody attributes now understood as single payer approaches. See D. Beauchamp and R. Rouse, "Universal New York Health Care: A Single-Payer Strategy Linking Cost Control and Universal Access," *NEJM* 323 (1990), pp. 640–644.

17. We refer to "traditional" Medicare in order to distinguish it from the Medicare plan that involves private sector HMOs.

18. See Steffie Woolhandler, Terry Campbell, and David U. Himmelstein, "Costs of Health Care Administration in the United States and Canada," *NEJM* 349 (2003), pp. 768–775. But see also Henry J. Aaron, "Costs of Health Care Administration in the United States and Canada: Questionable Answers to a Questionable Question," *NEJM* 349 (2003), pp. 801–803.

19. The catastrophic drug coverage program under Medicare that began phasing in on January 1, 1989, and was repealed, represents a program that was rejected in part because a vocal part of the population of beneficiaries believed they would be worse off with the benefit (after paying the required income-related premium) than without it. In many respects, the Medicare drug benefit enacted in 2003 is not as advantageous as the one that was enacted and repealed. This, and the fact that it is embedded in a more general and problematic Medicare reform, has led to strong efforts to correct the inadequacy of the legislation.

20. Marie Gottschalk, *The Shadow Welfare State: Business and the Politics of Health Care in the United States* (Ithaca: Cornell University Press, 2000).

21. In discussions about the Clinton proposal, which would have offered substantial benefits to firms that covered retired employees, Dr. Fein found that some firms that would have benefited were opposed to the proposal. The owners did not believe that the early retiree and other retiree provisions would survive the legislative mill, and thus the provisions as enacted (not as proposed) would not benefit them. Dr. Fein has also heard labor leaders privately concede the distributional inequity that arises from the failure to tax employee health insurance benefits. They are fearful of opening up a public discussion of

this matter, lest, whatever the details of the bill they started with, the changes made during the legislative processes would result in legislation that would harm their members.

22. See, for example, James Tobin, "Health Care Reform as Seen by a General Economist," Cowles Foundation Discussion Paper No. 1073 (New Haven, June 1994), and Michael Graetz and James Tobin, "Players and Payers," *New York Times*, op-ed (Feb. 11, 1994), p. A35, for a program similar to the one that we suggest. See also the following for proposals that are similar in some respects: Karen Davis and Cathy Schoen, "Creating Consensus on Coverage Choices," *Health Affairs*, Web exclusive (April 23, 2003); Victor Fuchs and Zeke Emmanuel, "The Universal Cure," *New York Times*, op-ed (Nov. 18, 2003), p. A25; David Cutler, *Your Money or Your Life: Strong Medicine for America's Health Care System* (New York: Oxford University Press, 2004). There is an extremely rich literature on numerous proposals, including a special issue, "Caring for the Uninsured and Underinsured," *JAMA* 265, No. 19 (May 15, 1991).

23. Ellen Meara, Chaplin White, and David M. Cutler, "Trends in Medical Spending by Age, 1963-2000," *Health Affairs* 23, No. 4 (July–August 2004), pp. 176–183.

24. It is also necessary to monitor disenrollment to make certain that delivery organizations do not behave in a manner that induces sicker patients to leave.

25. One could cover all children (thus reducing employer/employee expenses for dependents) or begin with uninsured children.

26. Roger Feldman, Kenneth E. Thorpe, and Bradley Gray, "Policy Watch: The Federal Employees Health Benefits Plan," *Journal of Economic Perspectives* 16, No. 2 (Spring 2002), pp. 207–217.

27. For political reasons Medicare beneficiaries might be excluded initially since they might be loath to give up a program they know works well for one with which they are unfamiliar. They could enter in a subsequent time period after the new program has demonstrated its effectiveness.

28. It is important that the level of premiums be adjusted in order not to provide an incentive for employers to drop health insurance coverage for their employees.

29. See Roger A. Rosenblatt, "A View from the Periphery: Health Care in Rural America," *NEJM* 351 (2004), pp. 1049–1051, for a discussion of rural health and the role of critical access hospitals.

30. This is true even though the Canadian system is one in which federal authorities set certain requirements and contribute fiscal resources, but in which the programs are administered and funded (in significant part) at the provincial level.

31. In an effort to deal with this set of issues, Dr. Fein advocated a series of state programs that would have received federal financial support. The participating states would be required to provide for universal coverage, but each state would be permitted to develop its own program and utilize whatever approach (for example, mandating or tax support) its representatives saw fit. While such a program had certain advantages over a single federal program, it suffered from certain handicaps. Among these was the fact that it was difficult to categorize the program since it did not fit into the existing descriptors (such as mandated, tax credit, tax-based, targeted). Nor did it deal with the problems that national employers with national contracts would face if the various states in which they were located elected different kinds of programs. See Rashi Fein, *Medical Care, Medical Costs: The Search for a Health Insurance Policy* (Cambridge, Mass.: Harvard University Press, 1986, 1989), pp. 193–222. See also Rashi Fein, "The Health Security Partnership: A Federal-State Universal Insurance and Cost-Containment Program," *JAMA* 265 (1991), pp. 255–258. This plan was endorsed by the Committee for National Health Insurance.

32. A governance structure analogous to the Federal Reserve System was spelled out, and considerable detail on the various responsibilities of such a scheme provided, in David D. Rutstein, *Blueprint for Medical Care* (Cambridge, Mass.: MIT Press, 1978). See also Donald L. Bartlett and James B. Steele, *Critical Condition: How Health Care Became Big Business and Bad Medicine* (New York: Doubleday, 2004), for an extensive discussion of health care and a suggestion that a Federal Reserve-like administrative and decision-making structure should be created for the health system. Consideration could also be given to the model of the Social Security Advisory Board, a seven-member independent and bipartisan board that advises the President, Congress, and the Commissioner of Social Security on Social Security matters. The Board publishes various reports and reviews. It does not have any operating responsibilities.

33. Also included, in addition to the fifty states, are Puerto Rico, the Virgin Islands, Guam, the Trust Territory of the Pacific Islands, and American Samoa. The various regions are headquartered in Boston, New York City, Philadelphia, Atlanta, Chicago, Dallas, Kansas City (Mo.), Denver, San Francisco, and Seattle.

34. Dr. Fein proposed this system to President Johnson's Task Force on Health in 1964. At the time other members of the Task Force were not convinced that the IRS could administer such a system. With greater computer capability this should not represent a problem.

35. The American Medical Association has presented a tax credit program. See Donald J. Palmisano, David W. Emmors, and Gregory D. Wozniak, "Expanding Insurance Coverage through Tax Credits: Consumer Choice and Mar-

ket Enhancements—The AMA Proposal for Health Insurance Reform," *JAMA* 291 (2004), pp. 2237–2242, and Mark V. Pauly, "Keeping Health Insurance Tax Credits on the Table," *JAMA* 291 (2004), pp. 2255–2256.

36. James Tobin in "Health Care Reform as Seen by a General Economist" presented a system of mandated individual enrollment that used the Internal Revenue Service. Tobin rejected employment-based insurance and provided a subsidy for the purchase of insurance that was roughly equal to the tax benefit middle-income individuals received because they did not pay taxes on employer-paid premiums on the employee's behalf. The program would have been financed by cancellation of Medicaid acute care (while retaining Medicaid nursing-home funding), elimination of the exclusion of employer-based health insurance from employee taxable income, and new cigarette and similar taxes (as called for in the Clinton program). The Tobin plan was not accorded extensive attention in part because it was presented as the discussion of the Clinton program was drawing to a close. It remains as a most significant (and generally unrecognized) contribution to the literature on universal health insurance.

37. See Julius Richmond and Rashi Fein, "Editorial: Health Insurance in the USA," *Science* 301, No. 5641 (2003), p. 1813.

Index

National Health Plan, 78
National Health Service (Britain), 36, 72, 234, 269n16
National Health Service Corps, 105, 182, 205, 285n51
National Heart Institute, 22
National Human Genome Research Institute, 189
National Institute of Child Health and Human Development, 266n11
National Institute on the General Medical Sciences, 266n11
National Institute of Neurological Diseases and Blindness, 22
National Institutes of Health, 3, 21–24, 27, 43, 99, 103, 160–164, 168–170, 172, 175, 182, 196, 217–218, 266n11, 272n15, 282n24
National Labor Relations Board, 38, 235–236
National Library of Medicine, 266n11
National Resident Matching Program, 206
National Transportation Safety Board, 166
Neighborhood health centers, 3, 45–46, 56, 186
Neurochemistry, 198
Neurosciences, 169, 194, 198–199
Newborns' and Mothers' Health Protection Act, 150
New England Journal of Medicine, 132–133
New Jersey, 208
New York City, 36
9/11 terrorist attacks, 166
Nixon, Richard M., 36, 46–47, 59, 63–65, 69–71, 76–79, 127, 135, 145, 155–156, 194, 230
North Carolina, 223
Nurse-midwives, 14
Nurse-practitioners, 104, 185, 226

Nurses Training Act, 56
Nursing/nurses, 13–14, 50, 68, 167
Nursing aides, 14
Nursing homes, 49, 130, 237, 294n36
Nutrition, 27, 91, 153, 163, 194–195, 203

Oak Ridge National Laboratory, 168
Obesity, 158, 195
Occupational Safety and Health Administration, 163, 281n17
"Off-shore" medical schools, 108–109
Oklahoma, 34
Open enrollment, 154, 253
Operating rooms, 83
Oppenheimer, J. Robert, 204
Optometry, 56
Organization for Economic Co-operation and Development, 92
Organ transplants, 158, 197–198
Outpatient care, xi, 38, 64, 69, 167

Pakistan, 107
Parkinson's disease, 198–199
Parkman, Paul, 58
Parran, Thomas, 162
Pathology, 9
Penicillin, 172
Pennsylvania, 208, 289n45
Pharmaceutical Manufacturers of America, 290n2
Pharmaceuticals, 205
Pharmacists, 13–14, 56, 167
Pharmacology, 9, 25
"Phasing" approach to universal health insurance, 78–79, 248–252
Phenylketonuria, 159, 196
Philippines, 107
Physician assistants, 104, 185, 226
Physician-population ratio, 9, 12, 103, 105, 185, 205, 225–226

Physicians, 13, 15, 25, 56, 68, 132;
geographic distribution, 9, 14, 92,
105, 122, 186, 203, 205; supply of,
12, 81, 103–110, 118, 185, 202–
203, 205, 225–226; specialization,
15, 19–20, 115–120, 122–123,
130–131, 139, 144, 181, 205, 224–
225; fees, 33–35, 46–47, 49–50, 61,
79, 104, 133, 143, 183, 209, 225,
267n15; income, 34, 64, 134; conflicts of interest, 61, 123, 132, 169–
171, 173–174; choice of, 66, 139,
143–144; advertising, 87; primary
care, 105, 116, 139, 183, 186, 224;
unionization, 134–135; malpractice insurance, 140, 208–214; work
issues, 203–208
Physicians for a National Health Program, 216, 290n14
Physicians for Responsible Negotiation, 135
Physicians for Social Responsibility,
217
Physiology, 9
Pittsburgh, Pa., 289n45
Polio, 160
Poverty/poor individuals, 58, 79,
105, 195; War on Poverty programs, 3, 44, 55–57, 186, 230,
268n5; Medicare/Medicaid, 5, 47–
49, 61, 156; at teaching hospitals,
17, 26, 101; uninsured, 41, 74, 82,
149, 239, 249
Premiums: insurance, 31–34, 36–37,
59, 63, 65–67, 78–79, 134, 136–
137, 141–143, 153, 157, 186, 226–
227, 230, 235–237, 241; Medicare,
47, 50, 155, 290n2, 291n19; malpractice, 209–214; for universal
coverage, 260–261
Prenatal screening tests, 159, 196–
197
Prepaid group practices, 31–39, 62–

69, 117, 133, 143, 153, 181, 226–
227
Prescription drugs, 43, 173; benefit
under Medicare, 50, 154, 289n2,
291n19; new, 136, 158, 166, 170–
171, 173, 201; advertising, 171;
costs, 186
President's Commission on Mental
Health, 286n2
President's New Freedom Commis-
sion on Mental Health, 286n2
President's Task Force on Health,
293n34
Preventive medicine, xi, 14, 62, 65,
67–68, 94, 153, 159, 161, 193,
195, 201, 217, 232–233, 259
Price controls, 59–60, 80, 87
Primary care physicians, 105, 116,
139, 183, 186, 224
Prior approval, 60
Professionalism, 15, 87, 174
Project on the Clinical Education of
Medical Students, 180
Promoting Health, Preventing Disease,
94
Psychiatry, 198
Psychotropic drugs, 43
Public Assistance, 17
Public health, 14, 17, 27, 56, 95–96,
158, 160, 181, 187, 194–195, 201–
202, 217, 280n8, 281n17; im-
provements in, 89–95; and health
policy, 162–167
Public health schools, 95–98, 121–
122, 151, 167, 201–202, 281n17
Public Health Service, 4, 17–18, 21,
90, 97–98, 162, 164, 258–259,
272n12

Race, 40, 58, 74, 92, 104–106, 121,
184, 186, 202, 232
RAND Corporation, 195
Randomized clinical trials, 151